Living With Dying

A Complete Guide for Caregivers

by

Jahnna Beecham & Katie Ortlip, LCSW

Starcatcher Press
Ashland, Oregon

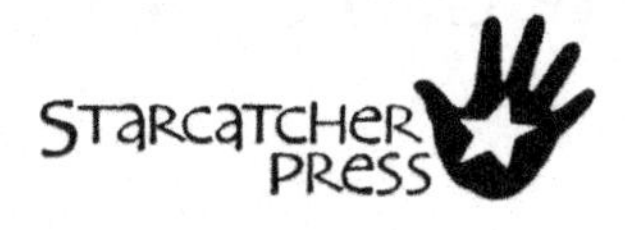

This book is not intended as a substitute for the medical advice of physicians. You should regularly consult a physician in matters relating to you or your loved one's health and particularly with respect to any symptoms that may require diagnosis or medical attention.

Printed in the United States of America

Living With Dying
A Complete Guide for Caregivers
ISBN 978-0-9973300-1-4 (pbk)
ISBN 978-0-9973300-2-1 (ebook)

Starcatcher Press
Ashland, Oregon
www.LivingWithDying.com

Cover Design: Jaimie Muehlhausen
Illustrations: Jack Wiens
Book Design: Maggie McLaughlin

For our children, Anna, Dash, Paul, and Skye—
so they can take care of us,
when the time comes.

Contents

Introduction vii

Part One: Living With Dying 1

1 The Journey Begins 3
The Emotional and Spiritual Voyage

2 What do We do Now? 11
Practical Matters

3 Traveling the Road Together 23
How to be with Someone Who is Dying

4 Taking Time for Yourself 31
Care for the Caregiver

5 The Way to Go 43
Hospice and Palliative Care

Part Two: The Caregiver's Manual 51

6 Setting Up the Home 53

7 Daily Physical Care 63

8 How to Care for a Bedridden Patient 75

9 Symptom Management 93

10 Pain—the Biggest Fear 123

Part Three: The Journey's End 137

11 How We Die 139
What to Expect in the Last Months, Weeks, Days, and Hours of Life

12 What to do After Death 153
Funeral Options and Who to Contact

13 How to Go on Living 161
The Grieving Process

Part 4: Resource Guide 173

Doc Talk 175

The 411 on Medications 179

WHO Pain Ladder 183

Online Resources 185

Suggested Reading 191

Index 193

Acknowledgments 199

About the Authors 201

LIVING WITH DYING

This practical, easy-to-use manual is for all of you caregivers who don't have the time to fix yourselves a meal or take a shower, let alone read a book. You who have so many health, legal, and daily care questions that you are utterly overwhelmed. You need help, but don't know where to get it or how to pay for it. Like you, I was in a constant state of high anxiety when my 90-year-old father was diagnosed with bone cancer. Unlike you, I had my friend Katie Ortlip to guide me through the final months, days, weeks, and minutes of my dad's life.

Katie is a former registered nurse who has been a hospice social worker for more than 20 years. When we were neighbors, she would often come home from work and tell me, "Today was a good death." I, of course, would pump her for all the details of what makes a good death because, in the end, that's really what we all want. Katie told me that most people want to die in their own bed, surrounded by loved ones, and just close their eyes and not wake up. But this doesn't always happen. Too often people find themselves in hospitals, on ventilators, hooked up to feeding tubes, surrounded by family members who are stressed at the doctors and arguing with each other. Everyone is in agony. Katie explained that this can be avoided if the patients make decisions about their health care ahead of time and choose a healthcare representative to speak for them when they can't.

I wondered if there was any kind of guidebook for dying and end of life care. Katie told me there were lots of books about love and loss and even the dying process, but they were often too wordy and time consuming for people to read in the midst of caregiving. Katie admitted that she'd always wanted to write a sort of "Death for Dummies" guidebook, because her patients and their families sorely needed it. Being a writer, I said, "Let's do it together."

We wrote this guidebook during my dad, Charlie Beecham's final journey. It offers practical "What do I do now?" information when you get the news, very specific caregiving techniques for feeding, washing, toileting, and communicating with your patient, and tips for taking care of yourself. Our guide walks you through the body's dying process and offers a road map for the physical, spiritual, and emotional journey you will take with your loved one. You will learn what I learned, and more. Because of Katie, I was able to be the best caregiver possible. And in the end, I wasn't afraid and Dad wasn't afraid.

He trusted me and I helped him. We laughed and sang together till the last hours. And on March 7, 2012 Dad had a good death.

Our hope, in writing this guidebook, is that by providing you with the knowledge and tools for end of life care, you will feel less afraid and more confident in your ability as a caregiver. And that you and your loved one will be able to savor every day, hour, and minute of life.

Jahnna Beecham and Katie Ortlip

Part One

THE JOURNEY BEGINS

ONE

THE JOURNEY BEGINS

The Emotional and Spiritual Voyage

Facing a terminal illness is an emotional roller coaster ride for your loved one, you, and your entire family. It begins at the moment of diagnosis when everyone knows that nothing will ever be the same. Navigating this new course can be bumpy as you weave your way through your grief. It's an emotional and spiritual journey that everyone takes one day at a time.

THE EMOTIONAL JOURNEY

Elisabeth Kubler-Ross, author of *On Death and Dying*, said grief has five stages that we travel through. Since her landmark book was written, other experts have said that we don't necessarily pass through all of these stages and sometimes not in this order. But it is helpful to understand them as a normal part of grieving.

Katie
I've had patients who were in denial the whole time, some who went back and forth from acceptance one day to denial the next, and some who couldn't let go of their anger. The same thing happens with caregivers. What's important is to be present, listen, and be respectful of each other whatever stage we are all in.

"Five Stages of Grief"

1. **Denial** is a normal coping mechanism that protects patients and caregivers from feeling too much pain too soon, before we are ready. Most forms of denial should be respected, and loved ones should not force patients to suddenly face their feelings. Give yourself, and them, time. Some may deny it until the day they die.

2. **Anger** is a common response of both the patient and the caregiver. It may be directed at doctors, family members, caregivers, and God. "Why me?" is the eternal question. Patients may become impatient and demanding. They can be downright mean to the ones they love the most. This can be extremely difficult when you are dealing with your own grief and are stressed out trying to be a caregiver and loving child or spouse. Keep reminding yourself that fear is driving this.

Katie
Some patients and families don't talk openly about dying because they're worried they'll upset each other. Grace, who had breast cancer, and her husband shared separately with me that they were worried that the other was in denial about Grace's prognosis. Once I assured them that the other did understand the situation, they were able to talk openly to each other.

3. **Bargaining** gives us a sense of control as we make promises or deals to allow us to live longer or make the whole situation go away. It's important not to crush a person's hope, but a caregiver should be careful not to lie about unlikely possibilities.

4. **Depression** is often described as profound sadness. It happens when the reality finally sinks in. Your loved one can go through bouts of crying, feelings of hopelessness, and withdrawal from the world. Though the sadness may remain, depression usually passes. If the black hole of severe depression persists, talk to your healthcare provider who can prescribe antidepressants. The same goes for you, who are trying to balance your feelings of grief, with the challenges of caregiving.

Katie
When I first met Barbara she was very depressed and cried the entire visit. The next visits weren't much better. Barbara felt stuck in her sadness. The nurse suggested she try an antidepressant, and within a week she showed improvement and actually smiled. She felt hope about the time she had left. Before Barbara died, she worked with a hospice volunteer to put together three photo albums as parting gifts for her sons.

5. **Acceptance** is the final stage. Though true acceptance is rare, most dying people come to peace with the facts by the time they go. Some people may not want to talk about death or even admit they are dying; yet they die peacefully. You may find yourself coming to acceptance as you watch your loved one's decline and want his struggle to be over.

THE CAREGIVER'S JOURNEY

The second your loved one is diagnosed with a terminal illness, everything changes. New roles are assigned to everyone and suddenly you are the caregiver. You might have done it before, for a few days or a week, but now you've been handed a full-time job that is both emotionally and physically overwhelming. As you take on this position you should know the givens:

- Your loved one's illness will never happen at a convenient time.
- You won't have enough time or money to help out the way you would like.
- Just when you think you've got all the caregiving solved, something will happen to make it all fall apart and you'll have to start over.
- You will probably quarrel with a close family relative about how to give the best care possible.
- At times you may feel overwhelmed by grief.
- There will be moments when you will probably feel resentment followed quickly by enormous guilt.
- You will start sacrificing your health for your loved one's.
- You might reach a point where you are burnt-out and absolutely certain that you cannot go one more day.
- Despite all of the above, in the end, you will be glad you were there.

Anticipatory Grief

Just as your loved one struggles to cope with his final journey, you too are preparing yourself for what you will do after he is gone. Your journey can be filled with anger, sorrow, and guilt. As a way of coping with the pain, you may find yourself detaching from your loved one and grieving his loss before it happens. This is known as anticipatory grief, and it is a natural reaction.

You may experience anticipatory grief so intensely that when your loved one dies, you feel numb. This can cause you to question your love, and yourself. All of this is normal. Anticipatory grief does not take the place of grief after death—that grief comes to each of us in its own way.

THE SPIRITUAL JOURNEY

Spirituality is difficult to define. It is about our connectedness to something larger than us; something beyond the physical. It is about life's meaning and why we are here. Spiritual care of the dying is as important as physical care.

Turning Inward

As our body dies, our world becomes smaller. Our thoughts move inward. Television, newspapers, letters, phone calls, and the constant chatter of the world around us become meaningless. Our lives are distilled to seeing and hearing only what matters most to us. There is nothing more important than this day. We should acknowledge this stripping away of non-essentials, and create a meaningful space where the dying person can find strength, inspiration, and hope.

FACING FEARS

Death is the great unknown, and our fear of that unknown is natural. We also fear pain and suffering, being a burden to others, and losing our dignity. Some patients fear being abandoned and dying alone. Others worry about what will happen to their loved ones when they are gone. And many are concerned that they are no longer useful to anyone. We have a few suggestions for addressing these fears.

Fear of Pain and Suffering

There are good medications that can help a patient stay as pain-free as possible. If you choose hospice or palliative care, the doctors and nurses can do much to keep a patient comfortable. See Chapter 5 (pg. 43) to learn more about hospice and palliative care, and Chapter 10 (pg. 123) in The Caregiver's Manual, to discover information about medications used to address different kinds of pain.

Fear of Loss of Dignity and Losing Control

The process of dying is a process of letting go. But it's important to let the patient have as much control as possible and to respect her feelings and wishes. Someone who is facing death doesn't want to be treated like a "dying person." Include her in decision-making, tell her what's going on, and respect her privacy. Filling out an advance directive is a good way for her to feel in control and direct her own care.

Fear of What Will Happen to Loved Ones

Some people fear more for those left behind than for themselves. This is especially true when the dying person has been the caregiver for a family member. This fear can be lessened by making a plan with the patient for what will happen to their relative after they're gone.

Katie

Linda was a 45-year-old patient whose biggest fear was how her daughter, who was developmentally disabled, was going to get by after her death. I connected Linda with a lawyer who worked with her to set up a trust for her daughter. Linda had a life insurance policy and set up the trust so Serena would get the money in intervals, rather than all at once. She also contracted with a case manager to look after Serena and manage the trust.

Fear of Abandonment

People tend to be isolated when they are ill and dying. Friends and even family members may feel uncomfortable and stay away. The patient may choose to be alone at times, but if she would like to have company, call friends and invite them to visit. Use computer apps, like Skype, to video conference. It's a good way to keep family members, who live elsewhere, connected.

Fear of Being a Burden to Family Members

The patient often feels guilty for the stress and burden he is causing others. He may feel bad for not taking care of himself or waiting so long to see a doctor. You can reassure your loved one that taking care of him is a labor of love, but you might want to take this moment to talk honestly about your own concerns.

If you are worrying about being able to manage his care and continue working, this might be the time to discuss hiring outside help, and ways to pay for it. Take the opportunity to problem-solve together. A working plan can ease both of your fears.

Fear of No Longer Being Useful

Much of the emotional and spiritual pain suffered by a dying person is from feeling a lack of meaning in his life. He may feel worthless because he is no longer "useful." These feelings can cause a deep despair. It's important for patients

Katie

Jim was a teacher and a master gardener before his illness. Confined to his recliner because of lung cancer, he complained of being useless and having no purpose in his life anymore. I began asking him for gardening tips and it became a part of our visits—me asking questions and him offering tips, and giving great advice about my garden.

to feel like they're still contributing. You might want to consider a life review, which is a look back at the highlights of his life. Here are a few ways to do it:

1. **Look through photographs.** Ask questions, label pictures. Find out the story behind the picture. Write it down. Create a "Best Moments" album together.
2. **Record your loved one telling stories about her life.** Make a list of specific questions: what was her best holiday, most embarrassing moment in school, first kiss, getting in trouble, scariest adventure, most fun memory of a sibling—all of these are great conversation starters. This interview can be a wonderful record for generations to come.
3. **Offer to write letters or make recordings.** Many patients have written letters to be given to their children at graduations, weddings, and the birth of their children.
4. **Ethical Wills** are documents or letters in which the patients share their values, blessings, hopes, life lessons and wishes for future generations.
5. **Host a Living Memorial.** This is a great opportunity to invite friends to come and celebrate your loved ones life, while she is still alive.

HOW TO ADDRESS UNRESOLVED ISSUES

Dr. Ira Byock, author of *The Four Things That Matter Most,* says, "I've lost count of the number of times I've met people in my office, an emergency room, or a hospice program who have expressed deep regret over things they wish they had said before a grandparent, parent, sibling, or friend died." In his inspiring book, he lists four simple statements that are everyday guides for doing the right thing, reconciling the rifts that divide people, and for resolving old history. These simple words are the keys to restoring closeness. They heal wounds and mend broken relationships.

The Four Things by Dr. Ira Byock

Please forgive me.
I forgive you.
Thank you.
I love you.

Saying Good-Bye

Dr. Byock points out that good-bye comes from the phrase "God be with you." Good-bye is not so much an end, but a blessed send off. We all want to say good-bye to our loved ones and let them know what a big part they have played in shaping our lives. They want to do the same.

Katie

Gayle's children had strong reasons for never wanting to see her again, but agreed to visit her one last time. Gayle was distressed. What she would say to them? So much had gone wrong in their relationship. I wrote Dr. Byock's "Four Things" on a post-it and gave it to her. When her children arrived Gayle gave them each a card asking for forgiveness and telling them she loved them. That opened the door for closure and Gayle was able to go in peace.

Two

WHAT DO WE DO NOW?

Practical Matters

The first weeks after your loved one is diagnosed with a terminal illness, you are in a freefall. You know things will be different, but you don't know how. You have so many questions, but the biggest is "What do we do now?" Some decisions need to be made and some subjects need to be discussed, but what are they? And who starts the discussion?

TALK ABOUT IT

Talking about dying is not an easy subject and each person handles it in his or her own way. Some patients and their families boldly face death head on. Others never want to admit out loud that they are going to die. But there is a middle ground where practical decisions about healthcare and caregiving in the coming months can be discussed. This is what medical professionals call, "Having the conversation."

The Conversation

There are things in life that are out of our control but each of us can face the future on our own terms. We can decide where we would like to spend our final days—at home surrounded by family, or in a care facility or hospital. We can decide what we would like to do with those days. We can choose what level of pain medication we would like. We can also determine what kind of procedures we want used to prolong our life and what kind we don't. And there is a way to make our wishes legal.

The Advance Directive

Doctors and hospitals in most states provide some kind of advance directive form. An advance directive is a great conversation starter. It's a form that allows a person to give instructions about final health care choices. You and other family members may want to fill out your own forms with your loved one. Forty-two states have a form they call the "Five Wishes" document. The document asks these five questions:

Five Wishes Document

1. What instructions do you want to give your physician about pain medications, medical treatments, and care, particularly procedures that will artificially prolong your life?
2. Who will speak for you about continuing or stopping those treatments when you can no longer speak for yourself?
3. How do you want people to treat you?
4. What do you want your loved ones to know?
5. Given that "doing nothing" would mean your comfort, care, and dignity would be assured, under what circumstances would you choose to forgo tube feeding or life support and be allowed to die a natural death?

https://agingwithdignity.org/five-wishes

As you fill out the advance directive with your loved one, approach each procedure with a hypothetical question like: "What if you had a stroke and couldn't talk—what treatments would you want?" Remind your loved one that having a signed advance directive means that her family and doctor will know exactly what she wants when she is unable to speak for herself.

Appoint a Health Care Representative

This is an important decision. The Health Care Representative is the person who will make sure that all of the decisions made in the advance directive are followed. This person is generally a family member and usually the main caregiver.

Jahnna
Dad, who was already getting demented, suggested his friend Joe from Kiwanis be his health care representative. I had to explain that Joe probably didn't know him well enough to take on that responsibility. He needed to maybe pick a family member–someone who would be by his side more often than not. My brother lived three states away and rarely visited. My mom was already overwhelmed by his care. He finally decided that I would be the right choice. (This is why it's a good idea to do it sooner than later.)

The POLST Form

A POLST form is the Physician's Orders for Life Sustaining Treatment. This form is signed by a physician and gives specific instructions to be followed by other health professionals. It reflects the patient's choices in the advance directive and is usually displayed on the refrigerator at home. All emergency personnel know to look there first before treating a patient. The POLST travels with a patient when he goes to a hospital or moves to a facility. Some states have a DNR (Do Not Resuscitate) form that gives instructions if the patient's heart has stopped and he isn't breathing.

LEGAL DECISIONS

A key part of your discussion with your loved one should include deciding who will be able to help manage her affairs, talk to doctors, and pay the bills when she is no longer able to do it. It is important to make sure your loved one is clear about what she wants done with her estate after she is gone. Decisions include: assigning power of attorney (POA), writing a will, avoiding probate, and creating a living trust.

Power of Attorney

This is invaluable for you as a caregiver. Basically, a Power of Attorney is a document authorizing you to take care of business and personal affairs for the patient. It doesn't strip the patient of her legal power, it just allows you to handle business—write checks, sign contracts, and buy and sell properties if necessary—when she cannot. It is a simple and inexpensive document that you absolutely must have. Get this sooner than later.

If the patient becomes mentally incapacitated, then she will no longer be able to sign a POA. And then you will need to go to court to get permission to become her legal guardian and that can cost thousands of dollars.

Once you and/or someone else have been assigned the power of attorney (it can be more than one person), a letter needs to be filed with the patient's doctors, bank, and anyone else you will be dealing with. It's also good to have your name put on the checking account and checks.

Durable Power of Attorney gives you the power to make decisions for the patient when she is physically or mentally incapacitated and can no longer make them herself. There are business and healthcare durable powers of attorney. It's good to have both.

Remember

Power of attorney and durable power of attorney are only for when the patient is alive. After death, you will not be able to write checks (unless your name is on the account), or sign contracts, or sell properties.

Guardianship

If a person can no longer make decisions or manage his affairs, and has not executed a durable power of attorney, a guardian (called a conservator in some states) may need to be put in place to protect the person's interests. The guardian can be a relative, friend, or a public official appointed by a judge. The process can be expensive and difficult. The best way to avoid this is for the patient to appoint someone he trusts as his durable power of attorney, while he can still make decisions.

Probate

Probate can be a long and drawn out process of making sure the will is valid, notifying potential heirs, and authorizing an executor to manage the estate. There are often piles of paperwork and thousands of dollars in legal fees, which in the end could eat up whatever money and assets were in the estate. It's not unusual for it to take a year or more. Imagine not having any access to your parent's cash, and being faced with having to pay the funeral costs, bills, house payments, and taxes until the estate is finally settled. Probate can end up costing between two and seven percent of the value of the estate.

How to Avoid Probate: a Living Trust

The Living Trust is a way of holding money, property, and other assets. It is a great way to avoid probate and have a smooth transition after the patient's death. If there is a trust, as soon as the trustor dies, bills can be paid, properties sold, and money distributed to heirs without going through probate or any court proceedings. Hiring a lawyer to set up a trust can cost between $1,000 and $2,000, but probate is more expensive.

No Need for a Trust?

Many patients avoid probate by putting their children's or spouse's name on their bank accounts, car titles, and house title. They divide their belongings among the family ahead of time.

What About a Will?

It's always a good idea to have a will, even if you have a trust, because odds are some asset has been overlooked and didn't make it into the trust. A will can list anything:

- Gifts of money you want given to friends or family
- Paintings or jewelry you would like a certain person to have
- Caveats about inheritance: "I would like to leave Jamie this amount of money to be used only to pay for college tuition."

The State's System

If you don't have a trust or a will, the state will distribute whatever assets you have after you're gone. If you are married, everything goes to the spouse, unless you have children from another spouse. Then everything is divided in half between your current spouse and those children. If you don't have a spouse, your assets are divided between your children. If there are no children, your parents will receive your property. If your parents have died, your brothers and sisters will receive your property. If you have no family, the state you lived in will get your property.

Important Papers

We should all have our important papers in one place. If they aren't in one place then there should be a list telling where the documents can be found. Consider getting a dedicated portable file box for your loved one's important papers. These include:

Personal Information

- Social security number
- Birth certificate
- Veteran's discharge papers
- Marriage certificate

Legal Matters

- The location of the will, if there is one
- The will's executor
- The patient's attorney
- The trust documents
- The safe location and key

Life Insurance and Death Benefits

- Life insurance
- Unions or organizations that provide death benefits, including phone numbers and membership numbers
- Retirement pay

Pre-paid Funeral Information

- Certificate for cemetery plot
- Receipts for pre-paid funeral home services

Real Estate

- Titles, addresses, and any important phone numbers of managers or co-owners

Banking and Stocks

- A full list of bank accounts: checking, saving, money market, IRAs, 401Ks
- Stocks
- Bank safety deposit boxes and key location
- Credit and debit cards

Taxes

- Recent tax returns and information for filing taxes

Royalties

- Publisher, agent, or company that distributes royalties for books, residuals for commercials and movies, and mineral rights

Automobile and Home

- Car titles and insurance
- Motorcycles, RV's, boats, titles, and insurance
- Home title and insurance policy

Phones

- Cell and home phone providers

Virtual Life

- Email accounts and passwords
- User name and passwords for social media, blogs, and websites

CONTINUING THE CONVERSATION

Not everything has to be decided at once. But just going over the Directive may open the door to ask other questions like:

- What are your hopes for the time you have left?
- Do you have a "bucket list"—all the things a person ever wanted to do before they "kick the bucket?" This list can include everything from sky diving, taking a cruise, visiting an exotic place like Machu Picchu or the Galapagos Islands, to riding horses on the beach at sunset, visiting old friends, or returning to a birthplace.

Katie

Steve had advanced ALS and was confined to a wheelchair. When he started to have difficulty swallowing, he decided that he did not want to go on a breathing machine or have a feeding tube. But he did have some wants for the last months of his life. He took his dream cruise to Alaska with his family, went to his daughter's wedding 3,000 miles away, and was proud to publish an article in a prestigious medical journal about living with ALS.

Including Children in the Conversation

Many of us are hesitant to talk to our children about death. We naturally want to protect them from pain, but death is a part of life, and we must teach our children how to deal with it. The following guidelines and answers to commonly asked questions might help you better support your child.

General Guidelines:

Give accurate information based on your child's age and experience. If he asks if the patient is going to die, you must be honest, but gentle, telling him that the patient's body is too old or too sick, and cannot get better. Reassure him that we don't die from most illnesses.

- It is best not to overwhelm a child with too much or too complicated information. Try to be sensitive to what the child can take in and understand.
- Keep an openness that encourages the child to ask questions or talk. Have special times that you spend with only her, perhaps looking at photos or drawing pictures to give openings for talking.

- Listen to and accept children's feelings. Share with them what you are feeling. If your child sees you crying, tell him you are crying because you are sad that your loved one is dying and you will miss her very much. Sharing your feelings gives him permission to share his with you.
- If the child has been dependent on the patient for care, as with a parent, reassure her that she will be taken care of.
- Allow and encourage children to visit, talk with, and touch the patient. Before the visit tell your child what the patient will look like, the medical equipment that may be in the room, and explain that the patient may not be able to talk or respond the way she used to, but she can still hear.
- Let the child participate in your loved one's care perhaps by reading or singing to her, or picking flowers to place by the bedside. A child should never be forced to visit, or made to feel guilty for choosing not to visit, a person who is dying.

Frequently Asked Questions About Helping Children Cope

My mother thinks I should have my five-year-old stay with her while my husband is dying because it will be too hard for her. I think she should stay with us. Is she right?

Even if a young child does not fully understand the implications of death, they are aware that something serious is going on. Sending your child away right now could increase her fear and anxiety about separation from you, especially since she will be losing her father. Ideally, she should be prepared for his death ahead of time, and being around while he is dying will help her understand and adjust to the loss. This isn't to say she needs to be home all the time. Overnights or time with your mother will provide a break for you and your daughter.

My son is seven. How much does he understand about his Grandma's health? He's also not showing much emotion.

Most children between the ages of six and nine are beginning to realize that death is final and that all living things die. But they still don't see death as personal, and feel somehow they can escape it. They may also be curious and ask a lot of questions. Not all kids cry or show emotion, and they may feel guilty that they're not. This does not mean they are not grieving. Answer his questions honestly and in terms he can understand. Let him know he can share his feelings with you, but don't pressure him if he doesn't want to.

My wife has less than six months to live. We have been pretty open with our teenage son, but he has been pulling away from us lately, and not wanting to talk about it. Should we be worried?

From about nine through adolescence, children begin to comprehend that death is permanent, and they too will die. This is already a time of many changes for teens, both emotional and physical. When they're facing a loss on top of this, it may make them especially confused and overwhelmed. It is normal for teens to withdraw from their parents and turn to their friends for the support they need. Keep communications open and let him know that you are there for him. Some communities have peer support groups for children with dying family members that have been found to be really effective. School teachers and counselors should be informed when a child is facing a loss.

FINAL ARRANGEMENTS

Some people will just not want to talk about death, or funerals, or memorials and you will know it. But you do need to find out if any arrangements have been made. A good way to ask about funeral plans is to say, "We should probably get all of your important papers in one place. Do you have any documents or wishes that we should know about?"

A more direct way to talk about final arrangements is to talk about your own wishes: "I would like to be buried in the family cemetery." Or "I'd like to be cremated and have my ashes tossed to the wind on the ocean."

If no arrangements or decisions have been made by your loved one, then you and other family members may be left to make the decisions when you are in the midst of grieving, and not necessarily thinking clearly. This is how gazillion-dollar coffins or over-priced marble memorial benches get purchased. These are needless expenses that can be avoided by thinking ahead.

Jahnna
I felt really lucky that Dad had already made arrangements with a local funeral home several years before. He'd pre-paid for cremation. He also had purchased and installed a headstone at the family cemetery in Oklahoma. He even had all of the information we needed in a small folder that included what he wanted read and sung at his memorial.

When you both feel comfortable, you might ask if your loved one has any special requests for a memorial. Again, always bring it back to yourself and what you'd like, so that it is a two-way discussion and not a pressuring of your loved one to make decisions that he is not yet ready to make.

Organ and Body Donations

Many of us already thought about this when we got our driver's licenses and marked the "yes" box for organ donation. But it's important to understand that people cannot donate major organs if they die at home. However, you can donate corneas, skin, and other tissues. For more information contact:

The Coalition on Donation • www.shareyourlife.org • (804) 782-4920

Whole Body Donation is a program that gives you the opportunity to donate your body to science. There is no cost. Many organizations offer this service. They come and get the body and when they are finished, the remains are cremated and returned to the family. Your loved one can die at home. He doesn't need to be in a hospital, and everything is free. There are some limitations so it is best to arrange in advance. For more information and a registration brochure contact:

MedCure • www.medcure.org • (866) 560-2525
MedCure accepts donations from all states within the continental US, except for Minnesota and New Jersey.

Science Care • www.sciencecare.com • (800) 417-3747
Accepts donations from all states in the US, except Minnesota and New Jersey.

CONVERSATIONS ABOUT DIFFICULT SUBJECTS

Many of the subjects discussed in this chapter don't need to be talked about immediately or ever at all. Appointing a health care representative and filling out an advance directive should be done soon. But take your time discussing funeral arrangements and memorials. You'll know if these subjects can ever be part of your discussion.

Right to Die or Death With Dignity

Most people don't want to die sooner than they have to, but there are some people who would like to control the moment of their death. They don't want to go through the last days or weeks of a terminal illness. There are also rare cases of patients whose symptoms can't be controlled to their satisfaction, even with the best hospice care. In some states, these people have the right to end their lives.

> **Katie**
> Requesting the medication does not mean you have to use it. Most of my patients who have asked to have the medications, never used them. They like knowing that they have some control over how they die.

At this writing, four states have enacted Death with Dignity laws: California, Oregon, Washington, and Vermont. Death With Dignity laws allow adult state residents, who are terminally ill, but mentally competent, to voluntarily request and receive a prescription medication to end their life. Montana allows physician-assisted death.

Hastening Death

As people come to the end of their lives, they stop wanting to eat and drink. Some patients choose to use this natural process to hasten their death by voluntarily giving up food and fluids. This helps them avoid suffering, and gives them control of their lives.

How it works: After the first few days of not eating or drinking, the body becomes dehydrated. The brain releases chemicals that act as painkillers and cause a euphoric feeling. Patients report feeling less pain than when they were eating. They don't have to go completely without water; their mouths can be moistened to quench the thirst. When the patient stops drinking and eating, it generally takes about one to two weeks to die. This can be a very peaceful way to go.

> **Katie**
> I had a patient suffering from Parkinson's disease. He was bedbound. His body was contracted. He was in worsening pain and having difficulty swallowing. He decided that he did not wish to go on living this way. Because of the way the Death with Dignity law is written, he would have to give himself the medication to be able to die, but he was nearly paralyzed. So he decided to hasten his death by voluntarily giving up food and fluid. The hospice nurse put him on a pain pump for symptom relief, and his caregivers kept his mouth moist with small sips of water. Within a few days he began sleeping most of the time and he died very comfortably in ten days.

THREE

TRAVELING THE ROAD TOGETHER

How to be With Someone Who is Dying

We all have questions about how to be with our loved ones, as their journey comes to an end. Often, we put on an optimistic face and pretend that they're going to live forever. We tell them not to be depressed or not to think about their prognosis. We do a lot of the talking, trying to avoid facing the bad news. This is a strain for both of you, as you try to keep up a brave front. When in reality, the single most important thing you can do for your loved one is to simply be present as you travel this road together.

How to Be Present

- Sit down, rather than stand over the patient. Sitting means I have time for you.
- Don't give advice unless asked, and resist the urge to cheer someone up.
- Allow your loved one to express regret. Don't say, "You've had a good life, you shouldn't be sad."
- To allow a patient a chance to open up, ask "What's your biggest worry or concern right now?"
- Accept people where they are. It's their journey and they need to move through it in their own way.
- Express love and appreciation openly.

Treat Your Loved One as a Mature Adult

- In the daily care, give your loved one as much control as possible. If she wants to take a bath in the evening and you prefer daytime, try to go with it.
- Be careful of talking behind a patient's back. She will think you are conspiring against her.
- Ask your loved one if she'd like to eat something now, and offer choices of food, rather than plopping a tray in front of her.
- Be very careful of talking about her as if she's not there.
- Be sure to ask the patient first if she'd like visitors.

Ask Questions

Jahnna
A month before Dad died, I ran into a woman who had recently lost her husband. We exchanged condolences and as she turned to leave, she stopped. "Be sure to ask questions of your dad—about his life growing up, his relatives, his best memories. My husband died and there were so many questions I wish I'd asked. Now I'll never know the answers." I went back to my parent's apartment and got out photo albums and started asking Dad about his life.

Listen

- Some people are anxious to discuss their deaths. Others never want to talk about dying. Let them know that you are there and ready to listen, but let them initiate that conversation.
- If you have to bring up a difficult topic, ask, "Is this a good time to talk about this? Or should we wait?"
- If the patient changes the subject when discussing a painful topic, that's your cue that she's done for now.
- If you need to discuss a tough subject and can't seem to be able to do it, ask for help from counselors or hospice.
- If you don't have an answer, say, "I don't know."
- Let your loved one express regret. We all have regrets about decisions we've made in life, and the pain we may have caused others. It's nice to be able to talk about them and have someone hear your "confession."

Seek Wonder, Joy, and Hope

The dying process is a series of little good-byes as the patient can do less and less, and we feel him slowly slipping away. Small pleasures become big joys. Sitting outside in the sunshine chatting over a cup of tea and a plate of shortbread cookies can be as special as any big event. Think of the opportunity to enjoy these small pleasures as a gift to both of you.

Katie

Time and time again, my patients tell me it's the simple things that bring them the most joy. One man remarked on the happiness he felt watching his grandchildren play in his yard and the yellow finches crowding the feeders. Another patient looked forward to cuddling with her daughter in her bed at night and watching old movies. Family members also learn to appreciate the simple wonders in life, and these moments shared with loved ones are what matter most.

Be Thankful

Katie

I often thank my patients for sharing with me their feelings and thoughts about their dying processes. I recently had a patient who openly talked about her emotional journey. During the first few visits, she cried about her feelings of deep sadness for having to leave her family and her daughter, who was pregnant. She shared what gave her life meaning—her work, family, and deep spiritual beliefs. During my last visits with her, she was in a place of such peace and lightness. On my final visit I found her dressed in a white gown, lying in her bed of all white sheets and pillows. She looked like an angel. I knew I wouldn't see her again and thanked her for all she had taught me.

Be Attentive to What Your Loved One is Experiencing

Many families and hospice workers report unexplainable experiences that have happened in their loved one's last days on earth. It is not unusual for patients who are dying to see people standing in the room or up in the corners of the room. They are most often visited by their mothers. Many reach dramatically toward an unseen person. It is common for patients to carry on conversations with their deceased friends and relatives, speaking, and then listening to their responses. Some events are truly remarkable. Pay attention. This may be an opportunity to get a glimpse of the other side.

- Mike had recurring visions of waterfalls and children playing. He told his wife, "If you could see what I'm seeing, you wouldn't be afraid."

- The last week of David's life, a flock of wild peacocks showed up at his house. Whatever room he was sitting in, they would be at that room's window. They stayed at the window all day and would roost in the trees at night. When he was dying, the peacocks stayed by his window until his death—then they disappeared.
- Ellie liked to feed stray cats and dogs, and kept her door ajar in case an animal needed help. When she was dying, animals from the neighborhood came to say good-bye. They were curled up on her floor, in chairs, and even on her bed.
- Katherine had two daughters, Betty and Amy. While she dozed, she kept visiting Amy, the daughter who had died. She would wake up and report, "Betty, I just saw your sister." Betty told her mother to tell Amy hello. Moments later, Katherine said, "Amy says hello back."
- Eight year-old Gabriel spent the last hour of his life lying in his grandfather's lap, wide-eyed and looking around the room, as if searching through crowds of people. Suddenly he sat up, smiled at someone or something in the corner of the room, then closed his eyes and died peacefully in his grandfather's arms.

Jahnna
My father told me "I'd sure like to see my daddy." (He had never called him Daddy before. It was always Pop, the nickname the grandkids had given him.) The night before Dad died, I slept in his room and listened to him having a lively conversation with his daddy. At one point he made a comment, listened, then laughed heartily and said, "I just knew you'd say that."

SPIRITUAL TOOLS

Spiritual tools can be anything that gives the patient peace and comfort. They also can provide an atmosphere of connectedness and closure.

Music

It is well known that music has soothing and healing powers. There may be certain sounds or pieces of music that touch patients on a deep level or just make them happy. Sounds from nature are also comforting—birds, ocean waves, rain. Harp and Native American flute music, hymns, chants, and classical music can all bring peace and joy.

Jahnna
Dad loved the song, "Bring Him Home," from the musical, *Les Miserables.* We played it over and over for him in his last few months. It became like a mantra guiding him to another life. He was listening to it when he died.

Meditation

Meditation is practiced as a way of looking inward and quieting the mind. To comfort both yourself and the patient, quietly repeat or sing a short phrase or scripture verse. Some examples are:

- "I am filled with light."
- "God, grant me peace," or "Dona nobis pacem."
- "The soul within me is pure."
- "I am held secure in the arms of love."

Conscious Relaxation

This can be effective in decreasing fears and anxieties. From what we know about dying, hearing is the last remaining sense. Dim the lights, light candles, play soft music, and speak in soothing tones. There are many relaxation tapes available, or you can try the following:

- Sit close to the person's head to be heard easily.
- Beginning with the feet, work your way to the top of the head, telling each body part to relax.
- Use as much detail as you want.
- Match your breathing with the patient's, and then slow your breath to see if she can follow yours.

Guided Imagery

In general, guided imagery is an imaginary journey that can lead to discovery and peace. In the case of the dying person, it can help with the transition. Although there are commercial resources available, you can easily be your loved one's guide by describing each step along the way, asking her to imagine the sights, smells, sounds and the feelings that go with them. Examples that some people have used include:

- A walk in the forest, through the mountains or on a beach
- Sitting in a lovely garden
- Describing what heaven might look like
- Visiting a favorite vacation spot

Massage

Touch has been proven to be not only healing and relaxing, but also helpful in pain management. The simple power of touch can be healing and comforting right up to the moment of death. Oils and lotions with scents can add to the soothing effects. Some frequently used scents are lavender, rose, sandalwood, and frankincense.

- **Foot Massage:** There's nothing like a good foot massage, and most people can tolerate them. Reflexology has shown that by simply massaging the foot we can ease pain and discomfort in other parts of the body. Massage the entire foot, including the top and sides. Prior to massaging the feet you can soak them in warm water.

- **Head Massage:** Position yourself above the patient's head with his head tilted back. Cradling the head with your fingertips, slowly massage the base of the skull, pulling your fingertips towards you. Gentle strokes with your fingertips on the forehead and into the hair and scalp can calm anxiety, relieve pain and aid in meditation. There are also pressure points on the ear. By using your thumb and index finger, gently rub the earlobe in slow, circular motions, working your way up the ear.

Create Rituals

For centuries people have been using rituals to help connect the physical life with the spiritual one. Rituals can be from religious traditions or personal to the dying and their families. Some simple ones are:

- **Candles:** Lighting a candle can signify a sacred time. Lighting a candle at the time of death can be very comforting at that moment of transition. The candle can be saved and used as a remembrance of the loved one on holidays and even the anniversary of his or her passing.

- **Smudging:** The Native American ritual of smudging is used to purify a space or room before, during or after a ritual. Small bundles of herbs are lit, and the smoke is gently waved throughout the room. Herbs most commonly used are sage, cedar, and sweet grass. (Smudge sticks can be purchased at health food stores.) Chanting and prayers may be recited at this time. After death, smudging is used to create a smoke path for the spirit to travel.

- **Incense Burning:** The sense of smell invokes strong memories and feelings, and can add to the sacredness of this time, before and after the death. Use cedarwood, eucalyptus, frankincense, lavender, myrrh, rose, or sandalwood.

Spiritual Readings and Prayer

Sharing favorite passages from the Bible or other inspirational readings can be comforting to the dying and their families. You may want to include a minister, rabbi, or priest for support. Some people's spirituality may be being out in nature.

Katie
Everett wished to die outside, in the woods above his son's home. He had been an artist and a naturalist, and spent much of his life in solitude out in nature. On his last day, his son carefully carried him up the path to a bed that had been prepared for him in the forest. Family and friends gathered around him. They built a bonfire, played music, and laughed and cried as they shared stories about Everett. As his breathing changed Everett's son knelt close to him and held his hand. Everett opened his eyes briefly and, with a smile on his face, let go of his final breath.

FOUR

TAKING TIME FOR YOURSELF

Care for the Caregiver

Flight attendants instruct you to put your oxygen mask on first before putting one on your child. There's a reason for this—you need to be alive to be able to care for your child. The same goes with caregiving—you have to be at your best to give your best. The good news is there are physical, mental, and emotional things you can do to stay as stress-free as possible. Follow them. They work.

TEN WAYS TO DECREASE STRESS

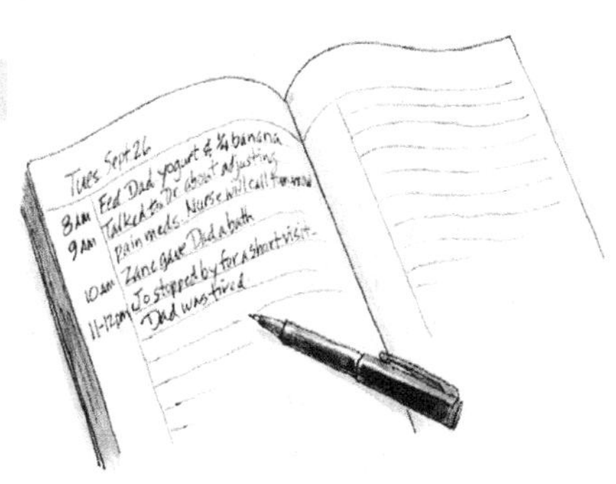

Step One: Keep a Notebook

From the moment you and your loved one get the news, start a notebook. You are going to be bombarded with information and unusual medical terms. Write everything down:

Doctors: Take notes at doctors appointments. You'll be amazed at how often you go back to them.

Medications: Keep track of what medications the patient is taking and update them as they change.

Phone calls: Keep track of every call to doctors, home care organizations, housekeepers, and insurance companies. Write down the date, who you talked to, what information you were given, and when to make a follow-up call. Even after your loved one is gone, keep that notebook. You will be making many calls. Having a clear record will be a big relief.

Step Two: Lower Your Expectations of Yourself

A new job has been added to your "to do" list. This will affect everything else. Acknowledge that. Really acknowledge that. Don't try to be super human. Let bosses, family, and friends know that your life will be different for a while. Cut yourself some slack. Know that your work output will be less at this time because you are doing a different kind of work. There is nothing wrong with you.

Step Three: Make a List of Your Loved One's Real Needs

This will help you identify what you do and don't need to do.

Jahnna

When my father was first diagnosed with bone cancer, I kicked into high gear trying to micro manage my parents' every move. It seemed like I was always criticizing them about food choices, hygiene, and their use of time. Finally, I made a list of my parents' real needs:

- A driver for grocery shopping, errands, hairdresser, and doctor.
- A liaison with hospice and doctors.
- A companion to talk to. This was the strongest need–the one that mattered most.

Step Four: Identify What You Can and Cannot Change

You can't change the prognosis of your loved one but you can make the journey a better one for you both. As you face the challenges that will come your way on a daily basis, ask yourself these questions: What can I change? What can I improve? What must I accept?

Step Five: Take Time

Time to breathe. Start the day focusing on breathing. Whenever you can, take five minutes to deep breathe. Use counts of five: breathe in through your nose on five, hold for five, and release through your mouth with your lips forming a shape like blowing up a balloon. This is a way to center yourself.

Time to gather information. You will be talking to doctors, home care organizations, and medical equipment people, and will have to absorb and understand a lot of new information. Allow yourself time for it to sink in. Make lists with pros and cons that will help you make decisions. A hasty decision usually results in having to make changes and more decisions. There are, of course, emergency moments, but most decisions can be given a little time—even if it's just to allow yourself the time to make a list of questions that you want to ask before you call a doctor or organization.

Time to eat right. You will be in a hurry to get home to the patient or to the doctors, pharmacist, or store. Sitting down to a healthy meal will seem too indulgent. It's not. Take the time to take care of yourself and make healthy food choices. Pack healthy snacks ahead of time in case you have to eat on the run. Just a little planning for what you will eat can make a world of difference to your wellbeing. Get a small cooler and keep food in it in your car.

Jahnna
I gained 17 pounds during my father's last year. Not because I was sitting in front of the TV with a gallon of ice cream, but because I was always so frantic that I never took the time to eat properly. My mom's pantry is always stocked with potato chips, chocolate, cookies, peanut butter crackers, and nuts. Those are her five food groups. And they became mine.

Time to exercise. Twenty minutes of walking or going to a gym will make you feel better. Think of yourself as being in training for a marathon, because that's what you're running when you are a caregiver. Keep yourself strong. Exercise is the best way to help you de-stress.

Time to do the things you love. Continue to sing in the choir or go to your art class—ask a friend or a volunteer to stay with the patient if he cannot be left alone.

Time to see your friends. It may be a diminished amount of time—an hour a week for coffee or lunch instead of the complete evening, but take the time. Combine the visit with exercise—walk and talk rather than sit and talk. Remember, your friends are your support system.

Time to just "be" with your patient. A lot of stress is caused by feeling like you have to be constantly doing something for your loved one. Many patients just like to have someone there with them. Sit and listen to music. Hold their hand. Don't talk. Just be.

Step Six: Keep a Good Mental Attitude

It's hard to avoid being in a constant funk when you're overloaded, rushing to carry in groceries and medical supplies, and dropping the papers you're supposed to fill out for doctors. All the while, your brain is screaming, "I can't do this. I'm overwhelmed!"

The best solution is to take a deep breath and think, "I can do this. I'll just take one step at a time." Take another deep breath. Think of three things that bring you joy: The autumn leaves, that dog happily playing across the street. A perfect latte. Stand up and clutch your hands behind your back and then release your hands. That gives you the best posture ever. Now, walk slowly to your loved one's door. Smile as you go in. It sounds silly, but these adjustments work.

Step Seven: Eliminate Guilt

Focus on what's working. "Please" and "Thank you" and a smile go a long way. Make a simple vow to say something nice to your loved one every day. Compliment her and tell her what a good job she is doing. Hugs are big. There are scientific studies that say a person who is touched and hugged at least once a day lives a longer and happier life. It doesn't take much to make someone's life better. You'll feel good. And so will they.

Jahnna
My guilt was huge. Quite often I was in such a big hurry to get to my parents, do errands for them, then get back to trying to keep up with my own life that I'd snap at Dad and especially Mom. I was frustrated that my 87-year-old mother wasn't on top of her game while taking care of Dad. (In reality I was distressed that my mom was falling apart, too.) I'd leave their house and immediately be slammed with a big, heavy weight of guilt. I was mean and I felt terrible. That guilt would keep me awake at night.

Step Eight: Reward Yourself

Sometimes it seems that nobody notices that you are working really hard and doing a fantastic job of juggling a zillion things. Then the resentment starts to build, especially against relatives who live far away.

People probably are aware, but not giving you the back-pats that you deserve. But don't wait for compliments. Instead, when you do something good, like make it through a week of caregiving, working, and taking care of your family—buy yourself flowers or a special bar of chocolate. Rent a movie just for you. Pour yourself a finger-full of that extra-special scotch, kickback, and listen to music. Find some thing or things that represent a present just for you. Make it a "celebrating you" ritual. You deserve it.

Step Nine: Ask for Help

Even if you are a Type–A personality, sooner or later you will surrender to the fact that you can't do it all alone. And that's a good thing. Though you may often feel powerless, you do have the power to ask for help. If you ask them, your friends will step up. If you let them, your hospice workers, hired caregivers, and volunteers from community organizations will become very strong shoulders you can lean on. You will also find this new village of friends and helpers will eventually hold a very special place in your heart.

- **Ask for help from friends:** People often don't ask their friends for help because they "don't want to be a burden." Friends are afraid to offer help because they "don't want to interfere." Ask for help. Friends help each other. Here's how to do it: Make a list of the chores that friends or family can do to help you and keep it on your refrigerator and in your purse. When they ask, "What can I do to help," show them the list. Always give them something they can do. If you don't, they'll think you can handle it and will stop asking. Your list might include:

  - ❑ Shop for groceries
  - ❑ Make a meal
  - ❑ Clean the house
  - ❑ Do the laundry
  - ❑ Sit with patient while you take time for yourself
  - ❑ Mow the lawn
  - ❑ Go to the pharmacy
  - ❑ Babysit your kids
  - ❑ Drive your kids to after school activities
  - ❑ Call your loved one once a week

- **Ask for help from family:** If you are the designated caregiver, but have relatives in the area, show the family the same list you show your friends. Ask them to make a weekly commitment to the item or items they have chosen on the *"I need help"* list.

Keep Friends' Phone Numbers in Notebook

Keep your friends' phone numbers in your notebook and make a note next to their name listing what they said they could do to help. Call them with specifics—date and time.

Your out-of-town family can also help:

- ❑ Visit and relieve you of duties for a short time.
- ❑ Invite your loved one to their home.
- ❑ Share care expenses.
- ❑ Hire someone to relieve you.
- ❑ Pay for a cleaner or gardener so you aren't overwhelmed by your personal chores.

If you have asked multiple times for help and they don't respond, let it go. Don't add to your stress by worrying about what those family members *aren't* doing.

- **Ask for help from your church or place of worship:** Religious organizations are champs at helping people who are stuck at home and overwhelmed by caregiving. Call them. They will also spread the word to the religious community who will mobilize and be ready to do what you need, even if it's just bringing a meal every week or stopping for a visit.

- **Ask for help from senior services:** These can vary from community to community. Many have respite or volunteer programs. Make the call. Ask what services they offer caregivers and their patients.

- **Ask for help from government agencies:** If your patient is a veteran, the Veteran's Affairs Office offers help.
  www.va.gov • (800) 827-1000.

If the patient is low income, low resource, and requiring care, he may be eligible for government help through his state Medicaid program. Contact your local Senior Services or Disability office.

Step Ten: Hire Help

If you are just overwhelmed and can't do it all, consider hiring caregivers to help you. They can be hired for just a few hours a day or round the clock. They'll do anything: give a bath, clean your house, baby-sit the patient while you shop, you name it. Caregivers can be hired privately or through an agency.

Your local senior services office will have a list of caregivers that have been screened for criminal backgrounds but it can be a tedious task finding one on your own. Agencies will do all of that work for you and also take care of taxes and insurance.

Hiring help can be costly if care is needed for a long time, but if you can afford it, it's worth it—even for small increments—especially if the patient wants to be home. (In Oregon, an average cost is $20 an hour through an agency and $15 for a private hire. Some agencies have a two or three-hour minimum).

Home Instead is a national home-care agency for seniors. To find one in your area: www.homeinstead.com (800) 640-3914.

Jahnna
If I had it to do over again, I would have hired caregivers immediately and started Dad's claim. He had Long Term Care insurance that required him to pay for his care himself for the first 100 days. We started it late and Dad died on day 99. Two years after Dad's death, Mom is still in shock about spending all that money for all those years and getting nothing.

How to Hire Help

- Determine how much help you need, the kind of help you need, and when you need it the most. Some people just need someone to come in for a few hours in the morning and a few hours in the evening.
- Decide if you want to hire privately (a friend with experience or one you get from a list) or from an agency. Private ones can be cheaper but caregivers from agencies are bonded, have liability insurance and have substitutes if yours can't make it.
- If the patient is on hospice call your social worker. She will be a great help in this area. If you hire privately, ask for references and check them out.
- Write out a mini-contract with the hours, expectations (be specific!) and the hourly rate.
- Call your Long Term Care insurance if you have it, and make a claim.

How to Manage Help

Make your expectations clear. Write a list. Think of it as instructions you might leave the baby-sitter. For example:

* Dinner at 5. Make Dad a salad with vinaigrette and macaroni and cheese. (Box is by stove. Salad ingredients in fridge.) Pudding or Fudgesicle for dessert.
* Bath at 6. Towels hanging in bathroom; fresh pajamas in the second drawer. Rub feet with lotion on the dresser.
* Dad likes to watch Turner Movie Classics.

* Toss clothes from today into the washer.
* When dad is watching TV, please wash dishes and clean kitchen counters.
* Clean bathroom after bath, and vacuum every 3 days.
* Put Dad to bed if he falls asleep in his chair for a long time.

What if Your Loved One Doesn't Want You to Hire Help?

"I don't want a stranger in my home," is the biggest reason given for not wanting to hire a caregiver. Remind your loved one that the caregiver will not be a stranger for long and hire one anyway. Explain that the helper is as much for you as it is for her. Just keep emphasizing the positives: "I want you to be able to stay at home. Hiring help will make that possible."

If you just can't get through to your loved one, it is very helpful to call in back-up–the doctor, a friend of the patient, a hospice nurse or social worker, or a mediator–to explain why hiring help is good for everyone.

How to Manage Conflict Between Caregivers

Hiring a caregiver is supposed to make your life easier, but it can be stressful if you have more than one caregiver and they don't get along. Right from the start, have the two meet each other. Sit down with them together and explain your needs and the needs of your loved one. Tell them they are part of your team and communication is the key. Explain that the goal is to make your loved one's life the best it can be. To make sure all your caregivers are on the same page, keep a notebook for them to record:

- Time of arrival—condition of the patient: happy, confused, etc.
- When and what the patient ate, and if she peed or pooped
- When the patient was given meds and when she slept
- Food or drink or any supplies that need to be restocked
- Any concerns the caregiver might have about anything

How to Minimize Family Conflict

- Review the patients wishes, keep the focus on what's important, so that your loved one can die in comfort and peace.
- Have regular family meetings and divide the labor.
- Don't let resentment build up, talk about it.
- Avoid using emails or texts to discuss important issues. This is where it all goes wrong. Talk face-to-face or through Skype or Facetime.
- When there is unresolved conflict, seek mediation.

The Battle at the Bedside

Since we began writing this book, we have met at least five people who are no longer speaking to any of their family members because of the fight over their parent's care. They argued over care facilities, caregivers, parent's belongings, and of course, bank accounts. Some of the parents had an advanced directive but no health care representative. This opened the door for siblings to go into fierce battle over what extreme measures should be taken for their mom or dad. One woman said, "When my mother died, I lost my entire family." Whatever the driving force behind these shattering fights, sometimes the only solution is to hire a health care manager to be an advocate for the patient.

HIRING A HEALTH CARE MANAGER

The manager will make the day to day decisions about the patient's care including: hiring caregivers, choosing a care facility, making the move to the facility, and making appointments with any medical professionals that the patient might need to see. They generally charge per hour but can accomplish a lot in that time. You can also choose what services you need from them. The Aging Life Care Association is a good place to search for all kinds of health care managers.

For more information: www.aginglifecare.org or call (520) 881-8008.

Note: Hiring a health care manager can also be a good solution if you live out of the area.

How to Care for a Loved One Who is not Loved

You may have had a terrible relationship with your parent but you get stuck with his or her care. You may have a brother or sister you can't stand, but you are the only living relative. Many people have to make the tough decision of whether or not to become the caregiver for someone they just don't like or love. Here are some tips.

- Be realistic about your limitations—what you're able and not able to do.
- Be very clear with the patient about your boundaries.
- Medicaid may pay for a nursing or foster home, or home care-givers.
- If you can't agree on care, hire a health care manager.

BURNOUT

Signs and Symptoms

Some of the following symptoms happen to most caregivers some of the time. But there comes a tipping point when you are so mentally and physically exhausted that many of these symptoms are happening all the time:

- Extreme fatigue—even when you sleep.
- Anger, constant irritability. Feeling resentful.
- Depression.
- Feeling like you're losing control—like you are going crazy. Finding yourself unable to enjoy life anymore.
- Becoming accident or illness prone.
- Entertaining thoughts of causing harm to your patient or yourself.
- Inability to concentrate.

What if You Just Can't Do This?

If your mental or physical health is suffering and keeping your patient in the home is no longer an option, here's what you can do:

- Understand that you are now harming yourself and make a change.
- Give yourself permission to stop.
- Forgive yourself.

What Should You Do?

Make a change. Start by talking to your doctor. She may prescribe medication for depression and/or refer you to a mental health professional. You also may want to include your patient's doctor in this discussion. He may be able to offer solutions by finding ways to help you get a break from caring for the patient or you may want explore care facilities.

Know that changing to a different living situation will be difficult at first, but your life will be better and so will your patient's because you will be happier and healthier.

Scary Fact

According to a 1999 study in the Journal of American Medical Association, if you are a caregiving spouse between the ages of 66 and 96 and are experiencing mental or emotional stress, you have a 63 percent higher risk of dying than people your age who are not caregivers. And if that's not bad enough, studies estimate 46 to 59 percent of caregivers are clinically depressed. This is why it's so important to take good care of yourself.

What Are The Options?

If your loved one is still fairly independent and you just need an alternative place where his meds can be given and meals prepared and there is someone around at all times in case he falls, you might be able to get him into an Assisted Living, especially if the facility knows that hospice is involved. But if your loved one is close to dying you probably want to get him into a skilled nursing facility or foster care home. If he has Alzheimer's or dementia, you might want to look into Memory Care facilities.

- **Skilled Nursing Facilities (SNF),** or nursing homes, are generally the highest level of care outside of a hospital. Aids help patients in and out of bed, bathe, dress and assist with feeding. There is a nurse on staff around the clock. SNFs will take terminally ill patients. The VA may cover the cost of a SNF of a veteran on hospice. To find the SNFs in your area: www.skillednursingfacilities.org

- **Assisted Living Facilities (ALF)** are for people who are fairly independent but may need assistance with activities of daily living. Aids are on call to help ensure the health, safety and well-being of residents. Some facilities allow families to hire a private caregiver. If your loved one is on hospice, this may make it more possible. To find the ALFs in your area, check out www.assistedlivinginfo.com or www.caring.com.

- **Memory Care Units** are facilities for patients with Alzheimer's and Dementia. They are more like a home environment than a skilled nursing facility and are better staffed than an assisted living facility.

- **Adult Foster Homes** (AFH) can be a wonderful option if they are available where you live. AFHs are private homes that are licensed by the state to care for around five people. They are rated by levels, according to residents' needs. A Level 3 foster home is licensed for total care and can take patients who are dying. Contact your local Senior Services office for a list of foster homes in your area.

- **Hospice Houses** are in-patient units where people can go when they are close to dying. They are not available everywhere. To find one near you: www.hospicefoundation.org.

FIVE

THE WAY TO GO

Hospice and Palliative Care

LIVING WELL UNTIL THE END

Simply put, if your loved one has a terminal illness, with a prognosis of six months or less, and no curative treatments are available or desired, there is no good reason not to have hospice. Hospice was established to provide comfort and dignity to patients and their families at the end of life.

As soon as you and the patient feel comfortable, talk to your doctor about bringing hospice into your life. A nurse and social worker will help you get the right equipment when you need it, work with you to manage pain and other symptoms, and help your loved one live the best life possible until the end.

Hospice Provides:

- A skilled team of professionals that includes: medical director, nurse, social worker, chaplain, therapists, home health aides and trained volunteers.
- Medications related to comfort for hospice diagnosis.
- Medical equipment such as oxygen, hospital bed, commode, shower chair, wheelchair, walker, and Hoyer lifts.
- Twenty-four-hour access to a nurse who will give advice over the phone, or make a visit if needed.

- Five-day respite in a skilled nursing facility for the patient so the caregiver can have a break.

- Some hospices have additional services like massage, music and pet therapists.

- Bereavement support and counseling for the family up to 12 months following the death of a hospice patient.

Jahnna
The first day Dad was put on hospice, a hospital bed, shower chair, toilet chair, and bedside table were delivered to my parent's home and set up and ready to go. And the hospice help never stopped. A hospice nurse took his vitals, filled his pillbox, assessed what was and wasn't working, and arranged for volunteers to visit and just to talk to Dad. If Dad needed a bed bath, a worker arrived to give him a bath. It's great to have a team that knows what you and your loved one have been going through and how to help.

Your Hospice Team

- **Hospice Medical Director** is a physician who works with your personal physician and the hospice team to manage the patient's symptoms and address new problems. They can make home visits as well.

- **Registered Nurse Case Manager** who will work with your family and the patient to develop, coordinate, and implement a care plan that maximizes patient comfort.

- **Medical Social Worker** will help you figure out care needs, financial and legal needs and can provide emotional support and counseling for the patient and your family. She can also help you access community resources like caregivers, alternative living situations and respite for the caregiver.

- **Home Health Aids** assist with bathing and personal care and tasks like changing the bed and starting the laundry.

- **Hospice Chaplain** is available to support the patient's spiritual needs. The chaplain can make home visits or will coordinate with your own clergy or spiritual support systems.

- **Physical Therapists** teach safe transfer techniques and how to use medical equipment. Speech and occupational therapists may also be brought in.

- **Trained Hospice volunteers** are available to provide breaks for caregivers and help patients with tasks like dog walking, shopping, light housekeeping, meal preparation, and general companionship.

SEVEN MYTHS ABOUT HOSPICE

Many myths are out there about hospice. Here are some of the biggest that Katie has heard and her response to them.

Myth #1: Hospice is a place where you go to die.
Hospice isn't necessarily a place; it's a way of caring for people. Most people have hospice in their homes. However there are some hospice programs that do have an in-patient facility or hospice house, usually for the final weeks of life.

Myth #2: Hospice means I'm at the very end and only have a few days left to live.
Not true. It is very difficult to predict how long someone has to live. While some people may die soon after being put on hospice, others are on hospice for months and even years. Actually, most of my patients wish they had gone on hospice sooner.

Myth #3: You have to give up hope and admit you are dying to go on hospice.
Hospice is more about living than dying. Although a patient is no longer receiving aggressive, curative treatment, her focus can now be on her comfort and quality of life. While people on hospice have terminal illnesses, they don't have to give up hope. Hope becomes about making each day as good as possible for whatever time is left.

Myth #4: Only people with cancer go on hospice.
Anyone with a prognosis of six months or less, who is not seeking curative treatment, can have hospice care. People with end stage heart disease, emphysema, Alzheimer's, neuro-muscular diseases and any end stage disease are eligible for hospice.

Myth #5: Hospice gives people "that shot of morphine" which kills them.

Hospice does not give drugs to kill patients. People are allowed to die naturally and hospice makes sure that they are comfortable and their wishes are respected.

Myth #6: Hospice provides 24-hour caregivers.

This is not true. The hospice staff (RNs, bath aides, and volunteers) makes routine visits. The nurse can come if there is an urgent need, but it's up to the patient or family to provide or hire the routine round the clock care that is needed. The hospice social worker can assist with finding caregivers or alternative living options if needed.

Myth #7: Hospice is expensive.

Medicare covers hospice one hundred percent. Medicaid and most private insurers also provide hospice coverage. Your local hospice can contact the insurance company to determine your coverage. If you are not covered, or uninsured, you will be charged on your ability to pay. Sometimes hospice provides free services. No one is refused hospice care for inability to pay.

QUESTIONS AND ANSWERS ABOUT HOSPICE

When can patients go on hospice?

To be covered by Medicare, Medicaid, and most health plans, the patient's health care provider needs to document that the patient has less than six months to live—if the disease runs it's expected course. Some patients live well beyond the six months. When a person goes on hospice they want to focus on comfort measures rather than curative treatment.

Katie

My patient, 89-year-old Ed, was rushed to the emergency room four times in three months with chest pain. Finally, after the fourth time, Ed's doctor asked him if he wanted to keep doing this, given that there was nothing they could do to fix the problem. Remembering the stress of calling 911 and the rides in the ambulance, not to mention the expense, Ed decided to stay home and have hospice care. The hospice nurse wrote out a protocol for what to do if he had chest pain. He could also call the nurse or me if he needed support. Ed never went back to the hospital and died comfortably at home.

Will I be kicked off hospice if I live more than six months?
Hospice does not automatically stop after six months. If you continue to meet the conditions for going on hospice in the first place—you have a terminal illness and you're not seeking curative treatment—then you can stay. Sometimes patients may improve or their illness has stopped progressing, and in those cases, they would be taken off hospice.

Should we wait for the doctor to suggest hospice, or should I bring it up?
The caregiver and the patient should feel free to talk with their doctor or health care provider at any time about hospice care.

Does a patient have to be homebound or bedbound to be on hospice?
Absolutely not. Hospice encourages patients to live as fully as possible, including taking long, wished-for trips, and spending time doing what they most enjoy. This is where the bucket-list comes in.

What does the hospice admission process involve?
After the patient's doctor orders hospice care, the hospice nurse will visit, assess the patient's condition and needs, and develop a plan of care with the patient and family. The nurse will want to address pain issues first and will work closely with the patient's healthcare provider to help the patient be as comfortable as possible. The social worker will assess the caregiver's emotional, social and spiritual needs. Other members of the hospice team can get involved as needed or wanted by the family.

Can I go off hospice if I want to try a new treatment? And is it possible to return later?
Yes. And yes. If your condition improves and the disease seems to be in remission, you can be discharged from hospice and even return to aggressive therapy if it's an option. You can always go back on hospice later.

Mom lives alone. Can she be on hospice?
Yes, of course. The hospice staff will monitor your mother's safety and ability to manage her own care. Hospice aids and volunteers can help with bathing and light housekeeping and meals, etc. When your mother can no longer live alone, the hospice social worker can help you and your mom look at hiring in-home caregivers or finding a foster home or a long-term care facility with 24-hour care.

I was told I shouldn't call 911 if my wife is on hospice. Is that true?
For the most part, yes. Most problems related to pain and comfort can be managed at home. And most hospice patients don't want aggressive measures. However, there are situations in which 911 may need to be called, such as a broken hip or a wound that requires stitches. Call hospice first, so your care can be coordinated.

What if my husband has a major problem in the night, like trouble breathing?
There is a hospice nurse available 24 hours a day. Most of the time the problem can be addressed by phone, but if needed, the nurse can come to your home, even during the night. The hospice nurse anticipates problems and usually has medications already in the home that can be used to address these problems, such as pain and shortness of breath.

What if my husbands' pain can't be controlled at home? Can he go to the hospital?
Yes. On rare occasions symptoms may be so severe that the patient and the hospice team will make the decision to take the patient to the hospital for a few days to get them under control.

Can a patient be on hospice if he hasn't agreed to sign a DNR (Do Not Resuscitate) form?
Yes. Under the patient self-determination act of 1991, a patient is not required to sign a DNR to have hospice care. However, each state enforces it differently. Be sure and check with your local hospice. Most patients do not want to be resuscitated since it is often painful and unsuccessful. Hospice is not required to pay for CPR. The family will be acting on their own if they call 911 for this purpose and may be responsible for the cost.

Can I have blood transfusions and still be on hospice?
Most hospices will cover procedures such as blood transfusions, thoracentesis (tapping fluid in lung space) and paracentesis (tapping fluid in the abdominal space), if they are for comfort. During hospice admission, patients should tell the hospice nurse what procedures they have been having and ask if hospice will continue covering them.

Does having hospice guarantee a pain-free death?
A pain-free death is never a guarantee, but your hospice team will be persistent in providing the best pain relief possible.

PALLIATIVE CARE

A common area of confusion is the difference between palliative and hospice care. Palliative care is comfort care. It focuses on quality of life and relieving symptoms (pain, difficulty breathing, etc.) related to life-threatening and chronic illnesses, such as cancer, heart, and lung disease. Palliative care can be provided for any person with a serious illness, whether the illness is terminal or not. The person can also be receiving treatment such as chemotherapy or radiation. Palliative care, like hospice care, is team-based care, including physicians, nurses, social workers, therapists and specialists, to provide comfort and support to patients and their families.

Differences between Palliative and Hospice Care

Treatment:

- Hospice provides care for the terminally ill with less than six months of life.
- Palliative care can be used alongside curative and life-prolonging care, and can be given to those with terminal and non-terminal illnesses.

Eligibility:

- Hospice patients must be certified as terminally ill, agree not to pursue curative measures, and elect to have hospice with a specific hospice organization.
- Palliative care patients must request palliative care referral from a physician.

Care Location:

- Hospice care is provided anywhere the patient is living (their home, a skilled nursing facility, a hospice house).
- Palliative care is sometimes offered by a care agency at home, but generally it is provided at a hospital, clinic, or care facility associated with the palliative care team.

Payment:

- Hospice and Palliative care are both covered by Medicare, state Medicaid, and private insurance.

If someone is in the last six months of life and is no longer wanting curative treatment, hospice is really the way to go. Though both options offer quality of life care with a multi-disciplinary team, hospice provides care in the home, and has bereavement support for the family later on. Hospice also has volunteers, and may offer such services as massage, acupuncture, music, and pet therapy.

For More Information on Hospice and Palliative Care:

Hospice Foundation of America
www.hospicefoundation.org
(800) 854-3402

National Hospice and Palliative Care Organization
www.nhpco.org
(703) 837-1500

Part Two

THE CAREGIVER'S MANUAL

Please Remember

This book is not intended as a substitute for the medical advice of physicians. You should regularly consult a physician in matters relating to you or your loved one's health and particularly with respect to any symptoms that may require diagnosis or medical attention.

Six

SETTING UP THE HOME

The goal is to keep your home as normal as possible for the entire family. Most patients want to stay in their own bedrooms as long as they can. When a patient is in bed most of the time, you may want to move him into the living room or family room so that he's not isolated and you can keep a closer eye on him. If the patient's bed is comfortable, let him sleep in it until the time comes that he needs a hospital bed. Care and equipment can all be adjusted as the patient's condition progresses.

Jahnna

Dad became obsessed with wanting to know the date and time, and asked about it constantly. We got him a clock with a large digital display and he was very happy. Later on, when he started asking where he was, I wrote a note and taped it next to the clock. It said, "This is your home in Ashland, Oregon. You live here with Norma."

Useful Items to Have Close to the Patient

- ❑ Small table by the chair or bedside, with water glass, tissues, lip balm, telephone, and small dish with pills that he can take as needed.
- ❑ Special blankets, candles, flowers, and favorite books can all bring comfort to the patient.
- ❑ Bell or horn to call for help
- ❑ TV and/or music player
- ❑ Favorite photographs and pictures
- ❑ Baby monitor
- ❑ Clock that displays the time and day

Fallproof Your Home

Falls are the most common cause of fatal injury in older people.

- Trip hazards: rugs, runners, bath mats, extension cords, space heaters
- Clear halls and stairways of clutter.
- Make lamp switches easily accessible. Add nightlights.
- Keep the telephone close to the patient's bed or chair, so it can be easily reached.
- Slip resistant rugs and runners can be purchased. Double-sided rug tape is also available.

Consider a Life Alert button for patients who are able to stay alone some of the time. They wear it around their necks and can push it to call for help if they fall or are in distress. The call goes to a switchboard operator who immediately calls to them over a speaker. That operator will call a family member, a neighbor, hospice or, if needed, an ambulance.

Fallproof Bathrooms

- Install grab bars in the shower and on the wall outside the shower.
- Put non-skid mats or abrasive strips in the tub.
- If the patient is unsteady, use a stool or shower chair.
- Attach a hand-held shower-head to keep everyone from getting wet.
- If the patient has trouble getting on and off the toilet, purchase a high-riser seat to place on the toilet seat or place a bedside commode over the toilet.

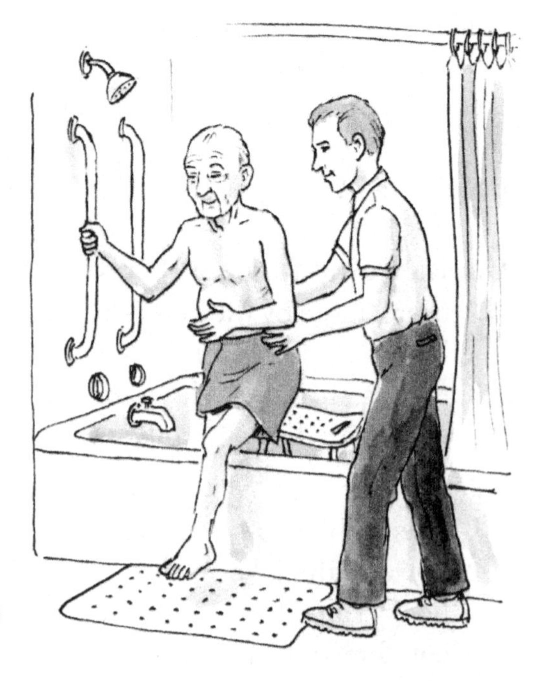

Fireproof Your Home

Burns are a leading cause of accidental death among seniors. Make sure you have working smoke alarms and an exit plan in case of fire. It's a good idea to have a transfer wheelchair, even if the patient doesn't need it yet, for a quick exit in case of fire.

- Purchase a fire extinguisher
- Keep candles, ashtrays, and smoking materials away from the bed or chair. (Don't let the patient smoke in bed.)
- Do not tuck in an electric blanket or place other covers on top of it—excessive heat can build up and cause a fire.
- Never set a heating pad or electric blanket on high.
- Never leave the patient asleep with a heating pad turned on.

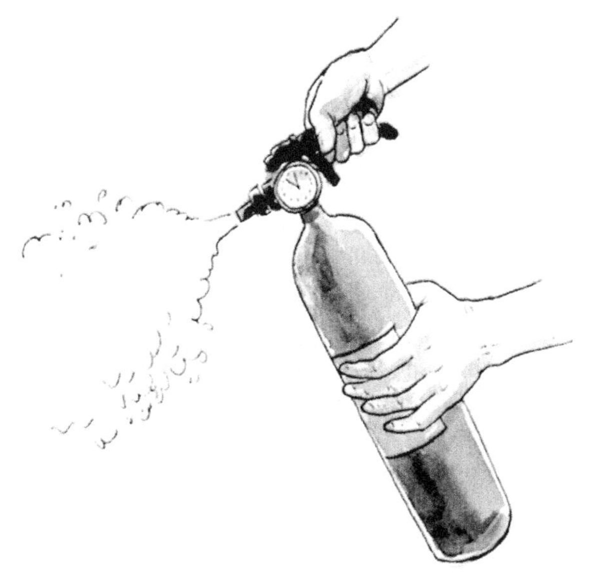

If you have to use it, remember P.A.S.S.—Pull the pin, Aim, Squeeze, and Sweep.

- As the patient gets close to dying, electric blankets and heating pads aren't advised because of temperature fluctuation and skin sensitivity in the patient.
- The stove can be a hazard if left on. If the patient is confused, consider removing stove knobs or protecting them with stove knob covers. There are many childproofing products on the market for making your entire kitchen safe.

Warning

Oxygen Feeds Fire. Do not smoke within 5 feet of an oxygen tank! Patients who smoked while wearing an oxygen mask have caught their faces on fire!

For Patients who are on Oxygen

- Oxygen should not be within five feet of candles, fireplaces, stoves, space heaters, or any kind of open flame.
- Keep a fire extinguisher close.
- Some patients' noses and throats get dried out from the oxygen, which can cause them to have a mucous build-up and sore nostrils. An easy solution is to add humidity to the oxygen. A water chamber attaches to the concentrator and the oxygen filters through it.
- Use only water-soluble lubricating jelly, like KY jelly, in the nose. This means no Vaseline petroleum jelly, Vicks Vaporub, or any kind of salve that contains oil or alcohol. They are flammable.
- Oxygen tubing should not be covered by bed linens, clothing or furniture.
- Be careful of tubing on the floor—it can be a trip hazard. Keep it away from any traffic paths in the home.
- All oxygen cylinders should be stored upright in a well-ventilated place.
- During very hot weather, cylinders should not be stored in cars or campers.
- Do not increase the liter flow of the oxygen without consulting your healthcare provider first. Too much oxygen can be harmful to some patients.

Lock Up Guns and All Weapons

Do this sooner than later. As patients get closer to the end, they may become confused or demented. This can translate into paranoia, distrusting loved ones, and thinking people are stealing from them. We have a friend who was discussing with his sister the need to lock up their father's guns the night before their dad shot his wife and himself.

Babyproof Your Home

- ❑ outlet covers
- ❑ stove knob covers
- ❑ cabinet locks
- ❑ grip and twist doorknob put medicine bottles out of reach
- ❑ furniture wall straps

THE RIGHT EQUIPMENT FOR THE RIGHT TIME

Good home care begins with safety and the right equipment. It's known as DME, or Durable Medical Equipment. DME includes a walker, wheelchair, hospital bed, swing table over bed, shower chair, bedside commode, oxygen, and any other medical equipment that makes the patient's and the caregiver's lives easier.

Who Pays for Durable Medical Equipment (DME)

If the patient has private health insurance or Medicare, a large portion of the cost is usually covered as long as the doctor orders the equipment. If the patient is on hospice, there is no need to call the doctor. DME is included in the hospice benefit and the hospice nurse will order the equipment for you and have it delivered to your home.

The Caregiver's Best Friend

The Gait Belt is a canvas belt that goes around the patient's midsection. It gives the caregiver something to grab onto when helping lift or transfer a patient. It can even be used in the shower or bath.

Walker

Some people prefer to use canes, but these may not be adequate as the patient becomes weaker. A walker is for patients who are unsteady on their feet, weak or prone to falls.

- Walkers with seats allow patients to carry things, and rest whenever they need to sit down.
- Instruct the patient to look straight ahead, not at her feet, to maintain balance.

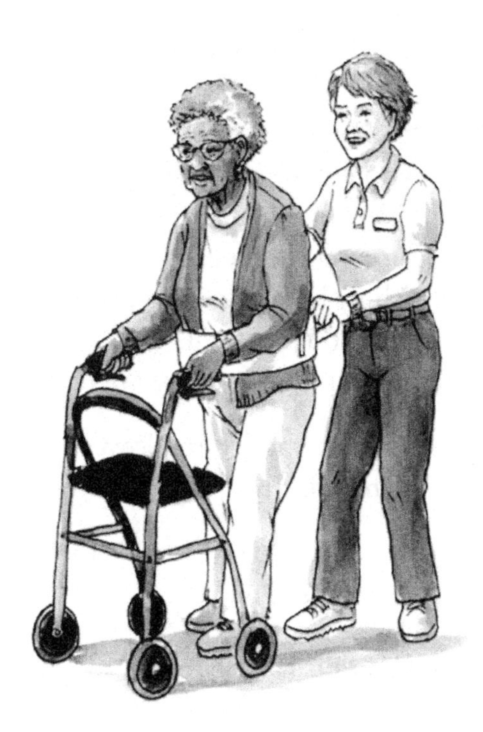

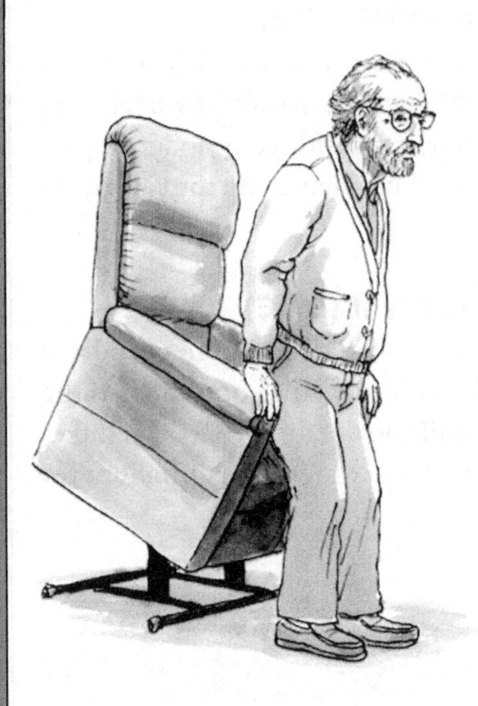

Electric Lift Chair

This chair looks like a normal recliner, but it actually helps the patient to a standing position. It has a simple controller with two arrows on it. If the patient has any confusion, it helps to write Up on the one arrow and Down on the other arrow.

Wheelchair

A wheelchair or transfer chair is for the patient who doesn't have the strength or is unable to walk. Most patients have transfer chairs (the ones without the big wheels) because they are lighter and easier to lift into cars.

- Lock the wheels of the chair before transferring the patient to or from a chair, bed, or car.

- Prolonged sitting in the chair may cause pressure sores to develop. An air or foam cushion will help prevent this.

Hospital Bed

Some people have a big fear of hospital beds. They think the bed signals the end. Hospital beds can provide great comfort to the patient as well as aiding the caregiver because not only do the head and feet go up and down, but the whole bed raises to waist-level of the caregiver. A raised head of the bed can help with patients who are having difficulty breathing. The patient is able to sit up and use a swing table for eating and other activities.

- Keep the bed in the lowest position when the patient is in bed. Then raise it, as needed, for care.

- Always keep the wheels locked except when you are moving the bed.

- Bed rails can be rented or purchased for a hospital bed and a regular bed.

Bed Rails are Controversial

Pros: Some people like bed rails because they keep the patient from falling out of bed. They offer a handhold for patients to reposition themselves and they can provide a feeling of comfort and security.

Cons: Patients have suffered serious injuries trying to climb over the rails or off the foot of the bed. If full-length bed rails are used, closely monitor patients who are confused or agitated.

One solution is to provide rails only at the head of the bed, from the elbows up.

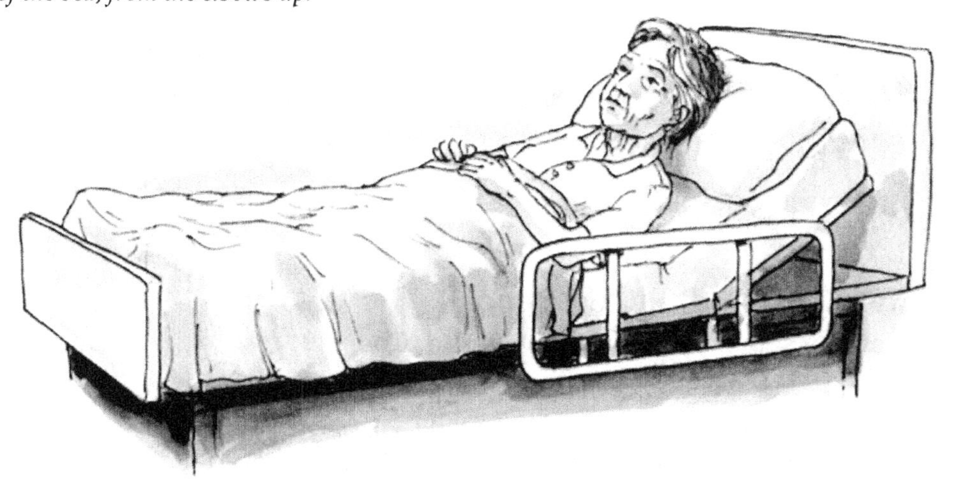

Sometimes patients with extreme dementia try to climb over the rails, which makes them extreme fall risks. If this is the case with your patient, put the box springs and mattress of a regular bed on the floor next to the bed, so they simply roll a few inches onto the floor and don't injure themselves.

Over the bed table

This is used for eating and activities in bed. It swings over the bed and to the side of the bed. It also raises and lowers as needed. It's very useful.

Trapeze

This can be installed over the bed and is for patients who want to use their arms to reposition themselves.

The Hoyer Lift

This is a hydraulic sling chair that safely transfers patients from the bed to the wheelchair or commode. It is for patients who are unable to bear weight and are just too difficult or heavy for the caregiver to transfer safely.

- A physical therapist or nurse needs to instruct the caregiver how to use it safely. (The Hoyer Lift is a useful option, but not necessarily a common piece of equipment.)

Bedside Commode

This is for patients who are too weak to walk to the bathroom or have to use it quickly and can be placed by the bedside or wherever the patient spends the most time.

- It can also be placed over the toilet. It has handles that help the patients push themselves to a standing position.

- It can be adjusted for height.

Shower Chair and Sliding Bench

These are for safe bathing in showers and tubs.

- The shower chair is a small bench (with or without back) that sits in the shower and can be adjusted for height.

- The sliding bench is good for homes that only have bathtubs. Part of the bench is on the outside of the tub, and part on the inside allowing the patient to slide safely into the shower, without having to step over the sides of the bathtub. It also can be adjusted for height.

Jahnna

In the five months that Dad was on hospice he used almost all of the medical equipment listed above. He went from a cane to a walker to a wheelchair and finally to a transfer chair in the house. We got him an electric lift chair, which he used as a bed, because it was more comfortable for his back. In the last week, he moved to a hospital bed and used the bedside commode.

Supplies

This list includes supplies for the patient who is incontinent and for patients who are confined to a chair or bed for most of their day.

- ❑ Adult pull-ups or diapers (buy a size larger to make sure they fit)
- ❑ Disposable gloves
- ❑ Bedpan
- ❑ Urinal
- ❑ Large disposable wipes
- ❑ Waterproof pads for bed and chair
- ❑ Hot/cool pack (We don't use heating pads any more because they can be dangerous.)
- ❑ Loose pajamas, nightgowns or large t-shirts that are cut up the back.
- ❑ Air cushion of foam pad for chairs to prevent pressure sores
- ❑ Egg crate mattress cover or air mattress
- ❑ Sipper cup
- ❑ Bendable straws
- ❑ Non-slip socks and slippers
- ❑ Lotions and creams for the whole body and lip balm
- ❑ Plenty of sheets to keep the bed fresh and clean.
- ❑ Plenty of pillows for helping position the patient in bed or a recliner—placing them under knees, between legs, and under the head.

SEVEN

DAILY PHYSICAL CARE

The caregiver's main focus should be on the comfort and safety of the patient. Symptom and pain relief are specifically addressed in Chapters 9 (pg. 93) and 10 (pg. 123). Here are five things you can do to give the patient the best care possible:

1. Prevent Falls

At first, a patient may be able to get around without any help, but as her condition progresses, this may change. Encourage her to use a walker, instead of a cane. It's more stable. Monitor her mental condition. The more confused a patient is, the more likely she is to take a tumble. Sometimes a bladder infection can cause patients to hold their body in a cramped position, which changes their gait and causes a fall.

2. Prevent Constipation

Offer foods that are easy to digest and include laxatives in the daily med plan if the patient is taking opioid pain medication. Remember, pain medications cause constipation!

3. Keep the Patient Hydrated

Place a cup with fresh water and a bendable straw next to the bed.

4. Focus on Good Hygiene

Cleanliness goes a long way to making a patient feel comfortable. There's nothing like a warm bath with sweet smelling soap and shampoo, followed by a body rub with lotion and the cool, minty taste of fresh-brushed teeth.

5. Keep a Daily Care Log

This journal is a great way to keep track of bowel movements, extra meds given for pain or anxiety and the time they were administered, and any new symptoms that appear. It helps the other caregivers and nurses track what has been done and allows them to determine if changes need to be made.

(Journal Example)

- 8:00 am: Breakfast: yogurt and small glass of juice. Ate 2 tsp of yogurt.
- 8:30 am: Took morning meds and dozed for an hour.
- 10:00 am: Complained of pain. Gave Percocet with good results.
- 11:00 am: Bowel movement. Large, soft formed.
- Noon: Didn't want lunch. Drank some water.
- 2:00 pm: Complained of nausea. Gave Compazine with good results.

FEEDING GUIDELINES

- Never force food or fluid on a patient!
- Five small meals are probably easier to eat than three big ones. And if the patient doesn't feel like eating, that's fine. Give patient the meals when they are pain-free and feeling good.
- Concentrate on food that is high in protein and calories for extra energy, such as protein shakes. Add Instant Breakfast to fruit juice or ice cream or make a high protein root beer float by adding vanilla-flavored Instant Breakfast and ice cream.
- When a person is nauseated, cool foods are best.

Katie
At this point in life, a person really can eat anything that sounds good. Chocolate shakes, cheese, crackers, cookies, you name it. Some of my patient's favorite foods have included biscuits and gravy, soft-boiled eggs, mashed potatoes and gravy, and every patients' favorite—chocolate mousse. It really is all okay. If it tastes good and doesn't upset the stomach, go for it!

- Meat is generally the first food that patients don't feel like eating, then veggies, and fruits. Don't worry about it. The body is doing what it's supposed to do.

- If a person is having difficulty swallowing: thicker liquids, like applesauce or pudding are easier to get down. Soups, shakes, puddings, ice cream, yogurt, and cool drinks seem to be the most appealing.
- Baby foods are soft and bland and can be appetizing with spices and seasoning.
- Crush flavored popsicles and offer little spoonfuls to help relieve the feelings of dryness when a person no longer wants to eat or drink.

FOOD FIGHT!

The most common struggle between the patient and caregiver is over food. The caregiver wants the patient to eat and the patient doesn't want to. This is a battle that you will not win. Some caregivers equate success with getting their loved one to eat a lot. Don't do that! Find another way to feel successful. Share a story, listen to music together, look through a photo album—these are all ways of giving love.

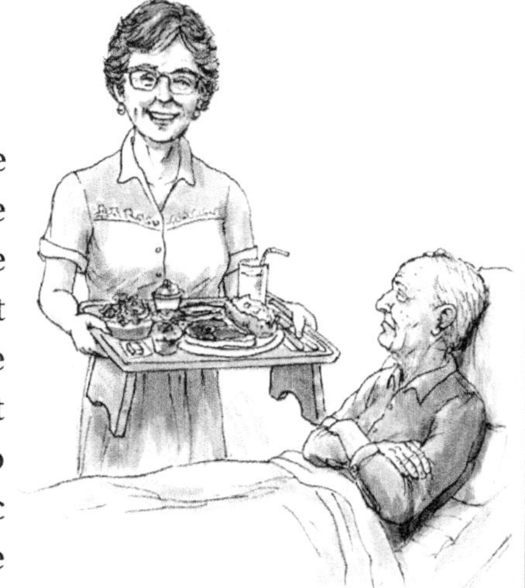

Don't force feed.

Why Won't They Eat? In General:

- Most dying people's bodies are in the process of shutting down.
- Their actual digestive system is not working as well as it used to, so the food can end up just sitting in the stomach for a long time, or moving slower through the intestine causing nausea and constipation.
- Meat is the most difficult food to digest, followed by rough vegetables, which is why patients reject them first and lean more towards soft, mushy foods.

Disease Related Causes for Not Eating:

- Patients with heart or lung disease are expending so much energy just getting their heart and lungs to work, there is little energy left for digesting food.

- Patients with advanced Alzheimer's eventually lose the ability to chew, swallow, and feed themselves.
- Cancer patients experience a change in their taste buds. They often complain that food no longer tastes good. Cancer is a force that robs the body of nutrition. So even when the patient eats, the body is not able to use the nutrients the way it used to. This causes weight loss.
- Patients with ALS (Lou Gehrig's disease) at first find it difficult to swallow, and eventually are unable to swallow.

Other Reasons for Decreased Appetite:

- Medications
- Nausea and vomiting
- Bleeding gums or mouth problems
- Weakness and fatigue
- Constipation
- Bowel tumors or obstruction
- Chemo and radiation
- Thrush
- Pain

THE FEEDING TUBE AND ARTIFICIAL HYDRATION

Though appropriate in some situations, feeding tubes or IVs are not recommended for dying patients who can no longer eat or drink. Here's why:

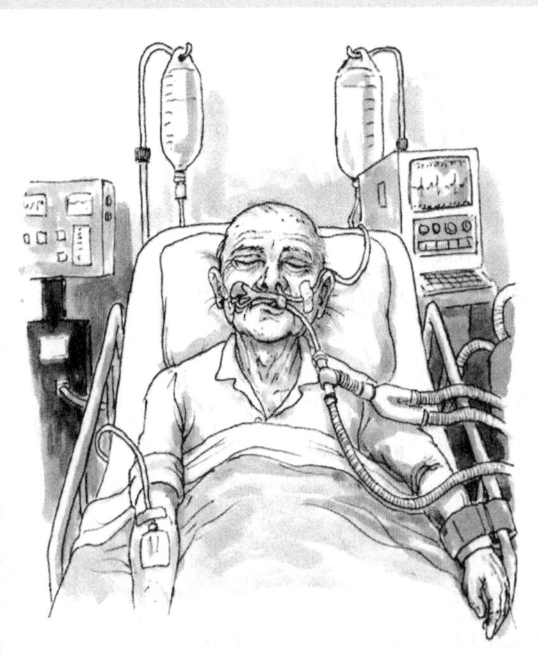

An Advance Directive could have prevented this.

- **They do not** increase the comfort of the patient.
- **They do not** cure the underlying disease.
- **They do not** prevent death.
- **They do not** offer a longer life for people who are dying.
- Forcing fluids or food will actually increase the patient's discomfort, because it will put an extra burden on the body that is no longer able to digest or deal with extra fluid.

Research Shows

As the body stops digesting food and begins to dehydrate, it releases pain-relieving chemicals that create an anesthetizing effect. Some have described the feeling as a "kind of euphoria."

GOING TO THE BATHROOM

Next to pain, elimination is probably the biggest issue for a patient. It can also be the most humiliating. Be sure you honor his privacy and treat him with dignity.

Staying Regular

There are a number of ways to make sure the patient has regular bowel movements:

- Laxatives should be included in the med plan.
- Movement of any kind keeps body processes going. If the patient can walk, a simple stroll around the room is good. Just the act of standing and sitting helps.
- Over the counter laxative pills or powders, like **Ducolax** or **Miralax**, can be mixed into juice or tea or administered in suppository form.
- Sometimes a daily glass of prune juice does the trick.
- **Smooth Move Tea**, which is made with the natural laxative, senna, is a pleasant way for a patient to stay regular. Stir in a capful of **Miralax** powder for extra help. Drink one cup a day. (Don't overdo it, otherwise you may face the other problem, diarrhea.)
- **Senna S** tablets are a mixture of stool softeners and stimulants.

Narcotics Cause Constipation!

Too many patients are started on narcotic pain medications without being put on laxatives. The two usually go hand in hand. The caregiver should make sure the patient has a bowel movement at least every 2–3 days. If constipation occurs, see Chapter 9 (pg. 104).

Going to the Toilet

Being able to use the toilet goes a long way in extending a patient's comfort and quality of life. Continue to take him to the toilet for as long as you can safely do it. When a patient is no longer able to walk to the bathroom on his own:

1. Use a transfer wheelchair to take him to the toilet
2. Using a gait belt, help the patient stand and pivot onto a raised toilet seat, or over the toilet commode.
3. Help the patient with his clothing and getting positioned on the toilet, then stand quietly outside the door (with the door slightly ajar in case he needs help or falls) to give him privacy.
4. If taking a patient to the toilet becomes too difficult, use a bedside commode.

Avoid Getting Stuck in the Bathroom

If the bathroom door opens inward and the bathroom is small, remove the walker or transfer wheelchair while the patient is on the toilet. Why? If he falls, the equipment could block the door and prevent you from getting in to help. Some people remove the door and replace it with curtains for privacy.

Daily Care of an Incontinent Patient

There are lots of comfortable and protective briefs that will keep patients from having any embarrassing public accidents. Most products and wet wipes are scented so there shouldn't be any worry about odor.

Jahnna

Dad wore adult briefs which looked like men's underwear and had extra padding in the front. We also added a Depend pad for extra absorbency. Because they were so absorbent, Dad only wanted to change once a day. We compromised by changing the Depend pad mid-day.

How to Use a Male Urinal

This can be used for patients who are bedbound or patients who have difficulty getting to the toilet.

1. Put on disposable gloves and place the urinal between the patient's legs.
2. Hold it low enough so that the penis can be inserted naturally into the urinal.
3. Leave the room, to allow the patient privacy.
4. When the patient is finished, empty the urinal and wash and clean with soapy water.
5. Give the patient a cloth to wash his hands.

The In-Dwelling Catheter for Women and Men

This is a small tube inserted into the bladder that continually drains urine into a bag. The tube is strapped to the thigh with a Velcro band and the bag hangs down by the side of the chair, wheelchair or bed. If the patient is still active, the tube can be attached to a leg bag that is strapped to the patient's calf. This is smaller and must be emptied more often.

Reasons for Using a Catheter:

- If a patient is incontinent, and he's getting sores from the moisture.
- If a patient is unable to empty her bladder.
- If a patient is completely bedbound and it's too difficult to change him, a catheter makes life much easier for everyone.

The Condom Catheter is Another Option for Men

- It slips over the penis and is secured to the penis with double-sided tape.
- The penis area should be shaved, so his pubic hair doesn't get pulled.

Katie

If a patient is demented or agitated and won't stop fiddling with the catheter, try putting an adult diaper over the catheter. If he continues to pull it out over and over again, it may need to stay out until the agitation can be controlled.

Catheter Care:

1. Clean the area where the catheter enters the body with gentle soap and water daily. Make sure the catheter is draining regularly.
2. If you don't see urine in the bag for a couple of hours, it could be clogged. Check the tube to make sure it's not kinked.
3. If the catheter tube irritates the bladder or is pulled out by accident, a little bit of blood may appear in the tubing or bag.

What to do if the Catheter is Pulled Out

If a catheter has been inserted for convenience, you don't have to rush to get it back in. If the patient has a catheter because she can't urinate on her own, a nurse or medical provider should be called right away. Either way, don't try to put it back in yourself.

Reasons to Call Health Care Provider or Nurse

- If patient has burning or cramping in his bladder area—it could be bladder spasms reacting to the catheter or infection. Drugs may be used to relieve spasms.
- If urine becomes thick, smelly, or cloudy with burning sensation—it could be an infection. Urine should be checked for an infection and antibiotics prescribed.
- Fever or chills—could be an infection.
- Large amounts of urine leaking around the catheter. The catheter could be clogged.
- Excessive bleeding (a little bit of blood is usually normal) could be a result of prostate or bladder cancer, or kidney stones.
- Swelling of the urethra around the catheter.

HYGIENE

How to Give a Bath/Shower

A daily shower or bath isn't necessary for the average patient. Depending on his needs, two or three times a week is a good number.

Before you begin, have all your supplies ready to go:

- ❑ soap
- ❑ shampoo
- ❑ towel and washcloths
- ❑ lotions

1. Make sure there is a non-skid mat in the tub and a stool or shower chair.
2. Close the bathroom door to keep the room warm, as you undress the patient, and put a towel or robe around him.
3. If a bath, fill the tub ⅓ full.
4. Help the patient into the shower or bath, keeping your hands around his waist. Have him sit on the shower chair. If there are handholds, encourage the patient to use them.
5. Be sure the patient uses the grab bars for support and not the soap dish or faucets.

Transfer Bench

A transfer bench stretches across the bathtub, with legs on the bathroom floor and legs inside. This chair eliminates the moment when a person has to transfer from the edge of the tub to the chair inside the tub. The person simply slides over.

Washing the Patient:

6. Turn on the water. Adjust the temperature and pressure away from the patient.
7. Offer him a washcloth to drape across his lap, for privacy.
8. Give him a soaped washcloth for him to wash his armpits and private parts.
9. If the patient ever feels faint, turn off the water, cover him with a towel, and have him put his head between his knees till he feels better.

Katie

We all shed dead skin, but elderly patients' bodies have a more difficult time sloughing it off. This can cause a build-up of scaly skin on their scalp, arms, and legs. Apply lotions often to soften the scales, the gently wash with a soft cloth. Never scrub.

Shampoo, Rinse and Dry:

1. If the patient is unable to shampoo his hair, have him tilt his head back and place a washcloth over his eyes.
2. A plastic sun visor works great for keeping soap out of the patient's eyes.
3. If the bathtub or shower doesn't have a hand-held showerhead, use a pitcher of warm water to pour over the patient's head to wet hair, shampoo, and massage scalp and rinse.
4. When he is completely washed and rinsed, turn off the water—away from him. Then help the patient out of the tub or shower.
5. Help the patient towel off, being careful to dry under the arms, breasts, and in all the skin fold areas. (Moisture can cause a yeast infection and rash.)
6. Dry the feet and apply any skin lotions to moisturize the skin.
7. Help the patient get dressed.

Mouth Care

Good mouth care is important, all the way to the end. You can use the patient's supplies that he already has on hand: soft-bristled toothbrush, floss, toothpaste, mouthwash and denture cleaner, if necessary. Have two glasses of water on hand—one to drink and swallow and one to swish and spit.

Mouth Care In the Final Days and Hours:

- **Toothettes** are sponges on sticks. Dip them in a glass of water and scrub the patient's teeth and tongue. It's a good way to offer water—the patient can suck on the sponge. Use the toothette every few hours to clean the build-up in the mouth and to hydrate the patient. Then apply lip balm to the lips.

- Squirt small amounts of water into the inside pocket of the patient's mouth. If they can't swallow, it will be absorbed into the gum and cheek. To keep the patient's mouth from getting too dry, add a drop of vegetable oil or coconut oil to the water. If the water causes them to cough, stick with the Toothettes.

- Dentures: Many patients don't want to be seen without their dentures, but as they get closer to death, they lose weight and the dentures don't fit. Sometimes they can cause sores. Ask if you can remove the dentures while the patient sleeps. Be sure and wash the dentures daily.

Jahnna
Dad loved brushing his teeth. I'd bring a soft toothbrush and a glass of water to his recliner and he'd spend a good ten minutes brushing. Even in the last days when he was actively dying, he liked the mint-flavored Toothette sponges on sticks. I'd brush them across his teeth and tongue and he'd suck on the sponge. I realized, even then, that there's nothing like the great minty feel of a clean mouth.

EIGHT

HOW TO CARE FOR A BEDRIDDEN PATIENT

In some ways, caring for a patient who is bedbound can actually be easier than transferring the patient in and out of bed. The number one concern for a patient confined to a bed is pressure sores. So here's a reminder of equipment you should use:

- ❑ Egg crate or foam pad if needed for comfort
- ❑ Waterproof mattress cover
- ❑ Extra flat sheets and pillows
- ❑ Incontinence pads
- ❑ Handle-held urinal for men
- ❑ Bedside commode for patients who are able to sit up and be transferred to the chair and back to bed again
- ❑ Adult disposable diapers with tabs

Patient's Clothing

The patient should be dressed in clothing that is comfortable for the patient and also easy for a caregiver to change. A lot of caregivers overdress their patients and often pile on too many blankets. People who are close to death often try to pull their clothes off. They just want to be naked.

Jahnna

Dad started out in the bed wearing sweat pants, a tee shirt, and sweater. We soon moved to the tee and sweatpants. Finally, he was wearing a T-shirt cut up the back and nothing else. In the end, Dad's body was so hot, we stripped him completely naked to cool him down and make him comfortable. We covered him with a light sheet. He looked like a baby being born in reverse.

Clothing checklist:

- ❑ An adult diaper with side tabs, instead of briefs. The adult diaper is easier to slip on and off and change when the patient can no longer help.
- ❑ It's easier with no pants, but if patient insists, use lose cotton pajama pants.
- ❑ Loose fitting cotton shirt or nightgown

SLEEPING POSITIONS IN BED

Pillows can help immensely with comfort for patients who are bed bound. The pillows relieve pressure on different parts of the body and help keep the patients safe and secure in the beds. Make sure you have a lot of them.

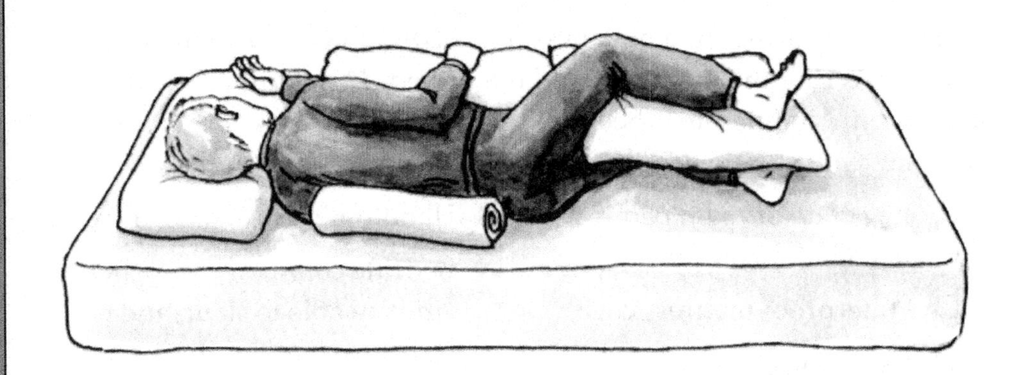

For a patient who has bedsores, but can't lie on her side.

You can place a small flat pillow below the area and one above, which will create a space and keep anything from touching the spot that hurts.

How to Move a Patient in the Bed

A draw sheet is the easiest way to move a patient in bed. It is simply a sheet, folded lengthwise, that is stretched across the middle of the bed under the patient's torso and buttocks and tucked in on either side of the mattress. One or two persons can slide the person toward the head, or the edge of the bed, by pulling on the sheet.

Using a draw sheet to move patient to head of bed:

1. Make sure the bed is flat and patient is lying on his back.

2. Remove the pillow and place it against the headboard to protect the patient's head.

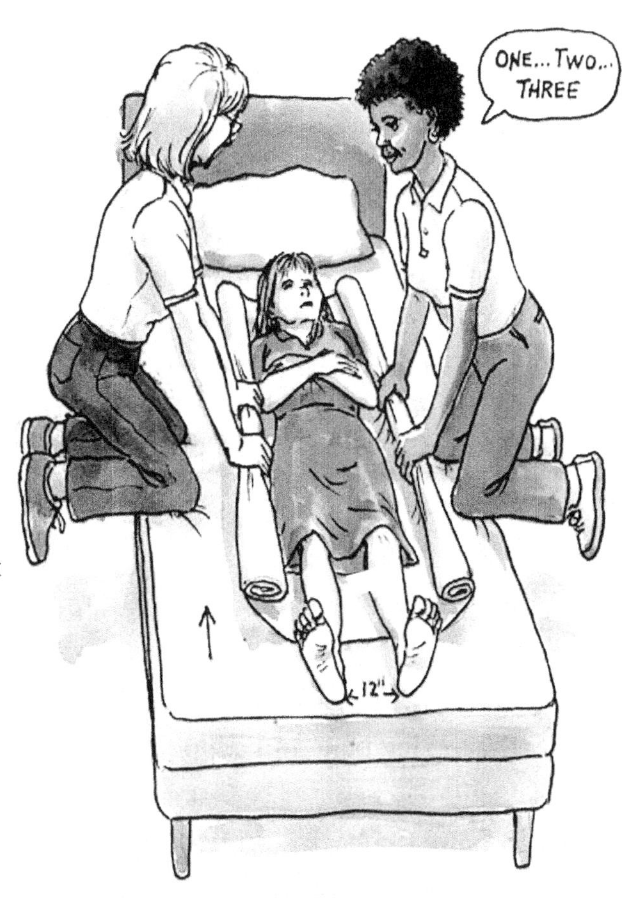

3. Un-tuck the draw sheet from both sides of the mattress.

4. If you are alone, bend the patients knees and stand at the head of the bed. Grab the draw sheet with both hands, as close to the patients body as possible. Bend your knees and pull.

5. If someone is assisting you, stand on either side of the bed. Roll the sheet to the patient's sides and grasp firmly.

6. Bend your knees and, on the count of three, slide the patient gently toward the head of the bed. (Always tell the patient what you are going to do, before you start moving him.)

7. Adjust the patient's body and put the pillow back under his head.

8. Be sure to smooth wrinkles out of the draw sheet and tuck it back under the sides of the mattress.

How to Turn Patient Onto Her Side Facing You:

1. Begin with patient lying flat on his back and have pillows nearby.
2. Make sure the patient is centered in the bed, so there will be room to lie on his side.
3. Cross the far leg over the leg closest you.
4. Cross the patient's arms across his chest.
5. Place one hand on his farthest shoulder and the other on his farthest hip.
6. Brace your body against the bed and roll the patient gently toward you using the draw sheet.
7. Check to make sure that the arm under the body is in front of the body with a bent elbow (not underneath the body).
8. Place a pillow snuggly along the patient's spine to keep him from rolling back.
9. Place a pillow under the head.
10. Support the upper arm with a pillow placed in front of the chest.
11. Adjust the patient's legs into a comfortable position with the top leg bent and supported with a pillow from knee to ankle.
12. Be sure the back is straight and the head is in line with the spine.

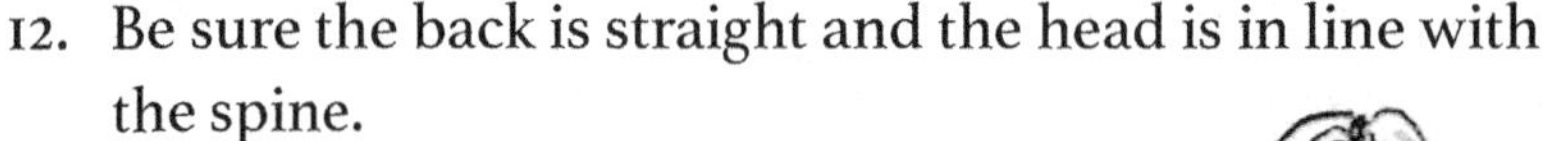

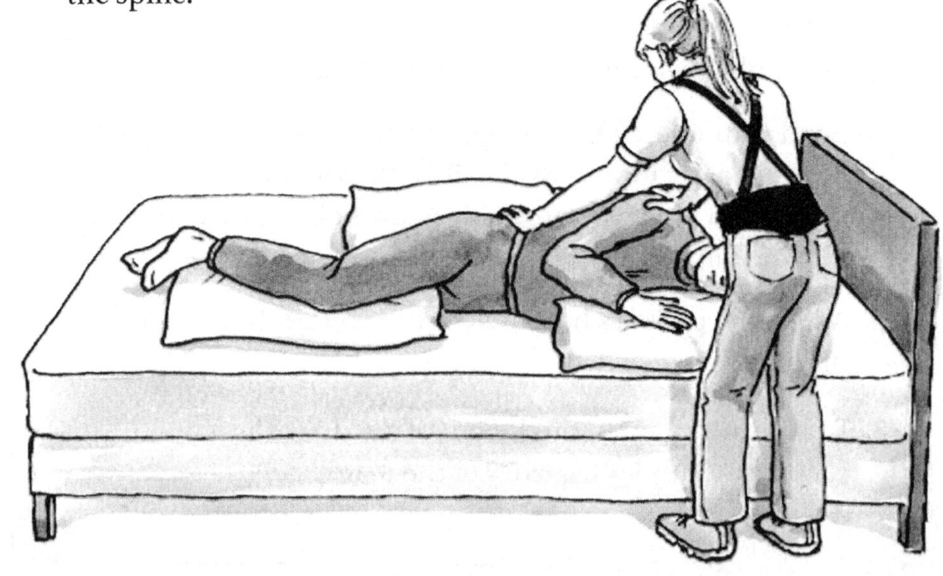

TOILETING A BEDBOUND PATIENT USING THE BEDSIDE COMMODE

Have ready ahead of time:

- ❑ rubber gloves
- ❑ toilet paper
- ❑ moisturized diaper wipes
- ❑ trashcan
- ❑ towel
- ❑ warm washcloths
- ❑ ointments
- ❑ clean diaper

1. Place the commode next to the bed.
2. Fill the commode with a little water, to make emptying and cleaning the container easier.
3. Move the patient into sitting position in bed and then stand them up and pull down their underwear or diaper. Then pivot him onto the commode. A gait belt will help you accomplish this.
4. Dignity is so important in all the care—as the patient sits on the commode, stand quietly outside the room. Or if the patient is in a big open living room, you might want to consider a privacy screen.
5. Be sure and provide toilet paper, wet wipes and ointment for the patient to wipe what they can.
6. Have the patient stand and wipe again if necessary, then help patient pull up underwear or put on a new diaper. Now pivot (taking small steps), and have him sit back in the chair or bed when he is finished.
7. Empty the commode in the toilet.

Save Your Back!

When transferring a patient to another chair or commode, stand as close to the patient as possible. Place one of your knees between the patient's knees. Bend with your knees and put your arms under the patient's arms and around her back in a hug. Instruct the patient to put her arms around you in a hug. Tell her, "On the count of three, stand." Then gently help patient to a standing position. Pivot patient to the commode by taking small steps, like a dance.

Using a Bedpan or Fracture Pan

Some patients like a bedpan—it makes them feel like they are sitting on a toilet. There are also smaller fracture pans that are less cumbersome and easier to use. But when patients are close to dying and cannot tell you they have to go, a diaper may be the most comfortable solution.

Gather Supplies:

- ❑ gloves
- ❑ toilet paper
- ❑ wet wipes
- ❑ washcloth and towel
- ❑ powder
- ❑ moisture barrier cream like **Calmoseptine, Vaseline,** or **Desitin**

1. Sprinkle a little cornstarch or baby powder onto the bedpan or fracture pan to keep the patient's skin from sticking to the pan.
2. Place a few drops of water or oil on the bottom of the pan and place a paper towel over that for easier clean-up.

Fracture Pan:

If the patient is able to lift up her bottom, the fracture pan is like a wedge that slides under the patient's bottom. For a patient who cannot raise her bottom, roll the patient on her side and press the fracture pan against her bottom. Then gently roll her onto her back, making sure the pan is in the proper position.

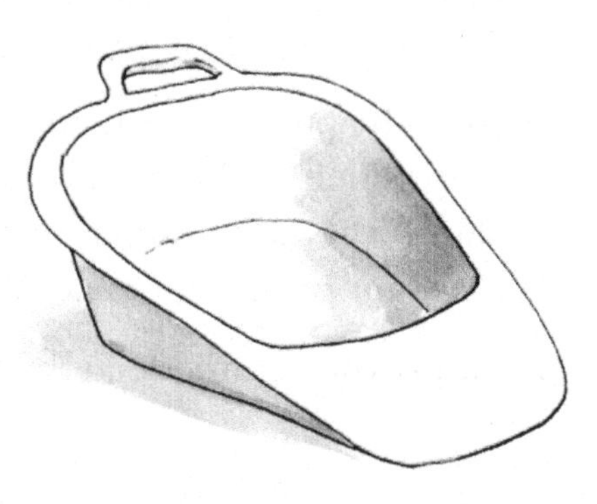

1. Raise the head of the bed so the patient is in a sitting position. Position pillows for extra support. For privacy, cover the patient with a light sheet.
2. If the patient is able to wipe herself, place toilet paper and wet washcloths within reach. Make sure you have an extra washcloth for the patient to wipe her hands.

3. When the patient is finished, lower the head of the bed.

4. Have the patient bend her knees and raise her hips if she is able and gently remove the pan. (You can help her by placing your hand under the small of her back and lifting.)

For the patient who is unable to lift her hips, roll her on to her side, remove the fracture pan and, if she isn't able to wipe, wipe (front to back) with toilet paper, wet wipes, washcloth, and towel.

Clean-up:

1. For a female, clean the area from the vagina to the anus with warm soapy water in a single stroke. Repeat process to rinse.

2. For male, clean the area from the scrotum to the anus using a single stroke. Rinse.

3. Pat dry and apply any creams that may be necessary.

4. Reposition the patient in the bed.

5. Empty the bedpan into the toilet and clean with soapy water and a toilet brush.

6. Remove your gloves and wash your hands.

Sometimes the patient is too confused or uncomfortable to use a pan of any kind, in which case, you can place an open adult diaper under her bottom, instruct her to bend her knees and try to poop into the diaper.

Remove Bedpan Immediately

Always remove the bedpan as soon as the person is finished using it. A bedpan can cause the first stage of pressure sores if left under the patient for more than 15 minutes.

HOW TO CHANGE A DIAPER OF A BEDBOUND PATIENT

If a patient is totally bedbound, pull-ups are no longer practical. You'll need to use an adult diaper with sticky tabs.

Before you begin, gather all of the supplies:

- ❑ Basin of warm water
- ❑ Gloves
- ❑ Toilet paper
- ❑ Disposable wipes
- ❑ Several washcloths
- ❑ Towel
- ❑ Moisture barrier creams for the skin and treating any sores
- ❑ It's best to get a diaper size larger than the person would normally use.
- ❑ Trashcan

Step by Step Instructions for Diaper Change

1. Open the diaper to see what you're dealing with. Clean the patient's front area first using TP, wipes and warm wet washcloth. **For women:** clean the labia area in the folds and wipe from front to back. **For men:** lift the penis and clean the scrotum and penis.

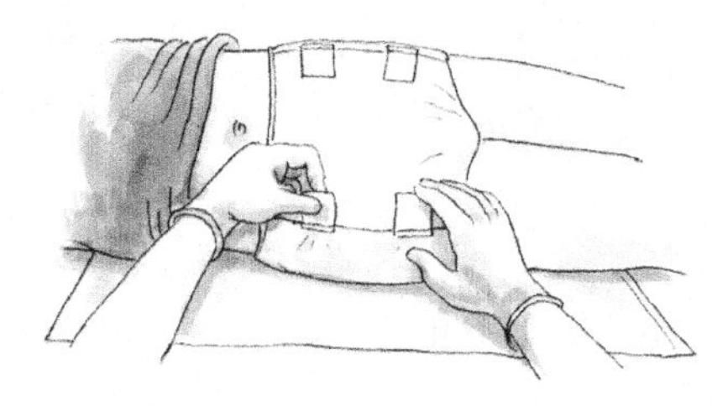

2. When the front is clean, turn the patient on his side. Prop pillows in front of him and against his back. Remove excess stool from the diaper and throw in the trash. Wipe, whatever you can off his skin with TP and wet wipes.

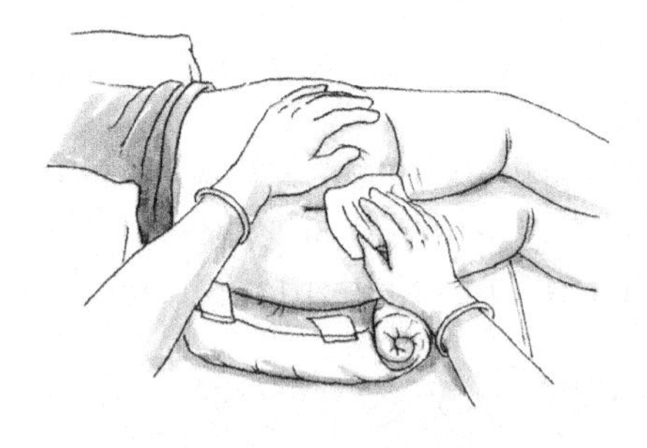

3. Roll the old diaper up to his body and tuck as much as you can under the body. Apply skin protection ointments and treat any sores.

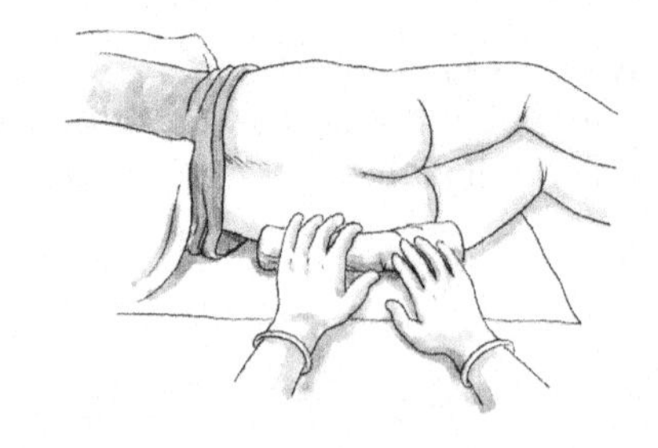

4. Turn patient to the other side, prop with pillows, and repeat the same process: Remove excess stool, wipe with TP and wet wipes, and warm wash-cloth.

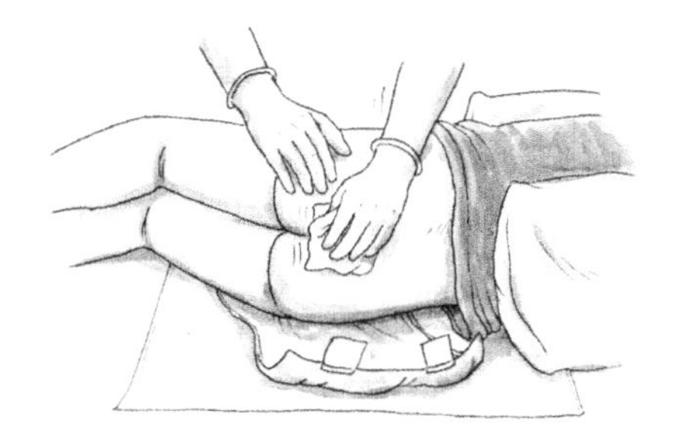

5. Roll up the rest of the dirty diaper and throw in trash.

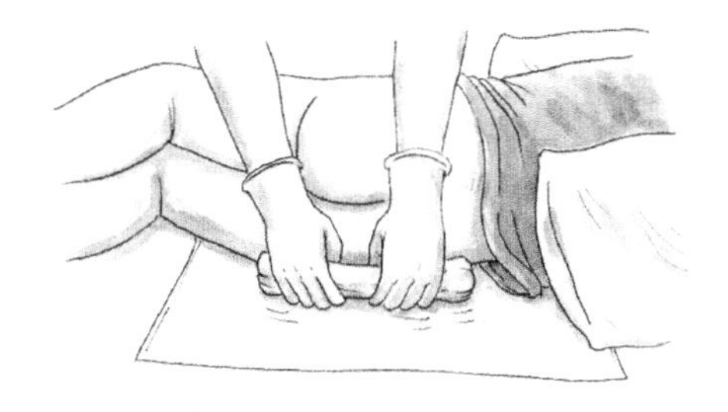

6. Make sure everything is clean and apply any creams that are necessary. If the patients has bedsores, place a piece of Saran Wrap over any creams that you've applied to the sores. That keeps the cream from rubbing off on the diaper.

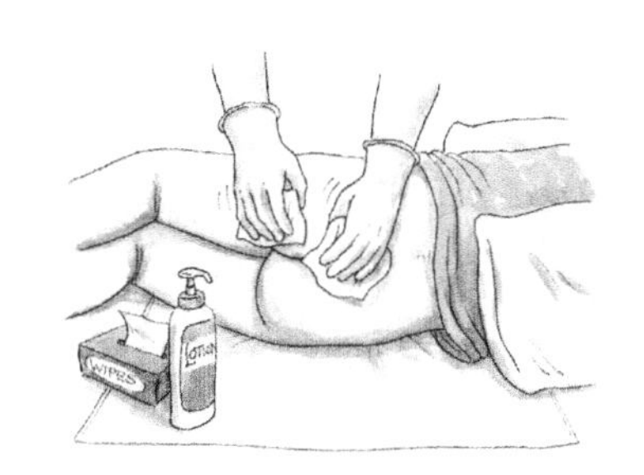

7. Press the new open diaper against the patient's bottom. Make sure the part with the tabs is at the top.

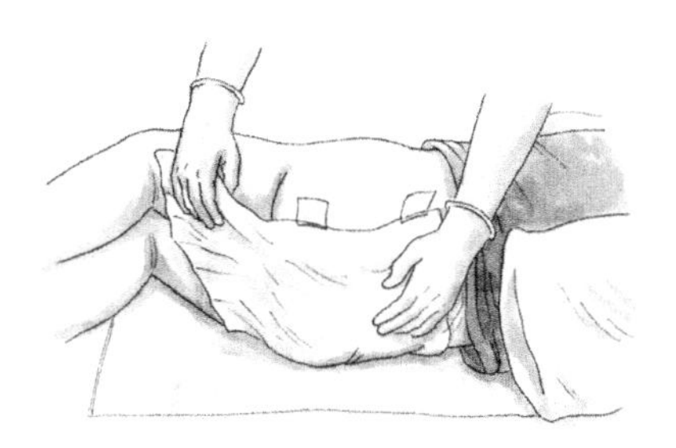

8. Gently roll the patient onto his back, smooth the diaper so that there are no wrinkles, and attach the tabs. If patient has a catheter, you can sometimes leave the diaper open. Otherwise close the diaper and attach tabs.

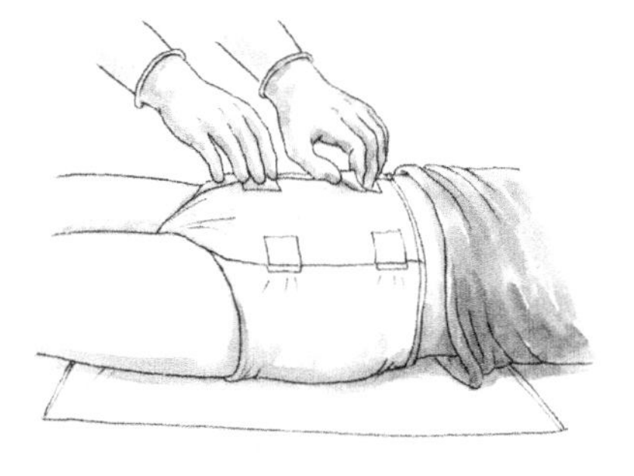

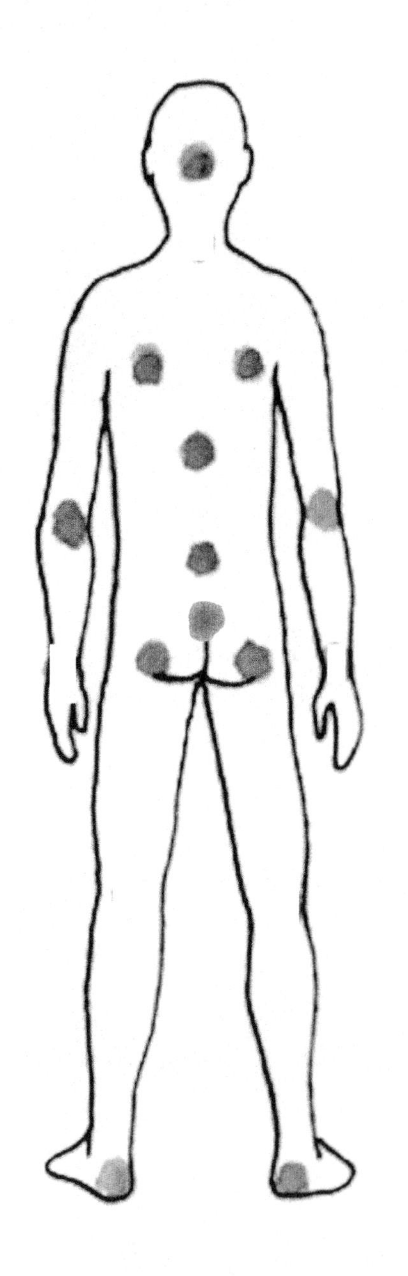

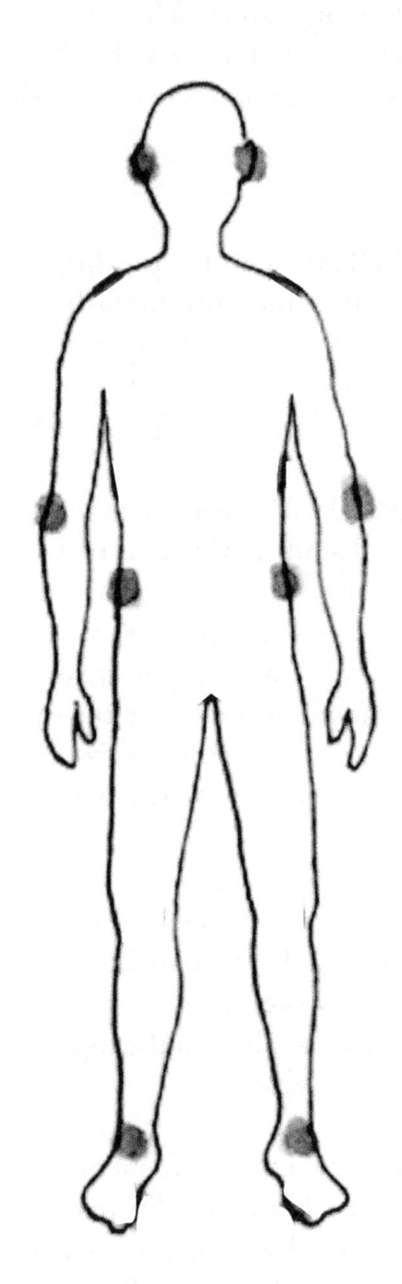

BONY AREAS MOST PRONE TO BED SORES

HOW TO AVOID PRESSURE SORES/BED SORES

The Best Treatment Is Prevention:

- Place air or foam cushions on chairs.
- Put an air or foam mattress top on the bed if needed.
- To keep skin from touching skin, use pillows. Put one between the legs, between the knees when lying on the side, under calves so that heels don't touch the bed. Put a rolled up towel between the arms and the body.
- Make sure sheets are wrinkle-free and dry.
- Change sheets when dirty, wet, or sweaty.
- The patient should move or be moved every 4 hours.
- If the patient is immobile, the caregiver can turn her with a draw sheet (see pg. 76).
- If a bed-bound patient can sit up and dangle his legs over the side of the bed several times a day, that will increase circulation.
- Add protein to the diet by mixing protein powder into drinks or shakes. **Vitamin C** helps healing.
- Use bath time to check the skin for red areas.
- Avoid using hot water. Use soap sparingly. Dry thoroughly after bath.
- Red areas, small breaks in the skin or hard to reach places between the buttocks can develop rash. **Calmoseptine** is a good moisture barrier that can protect the skin. Other diaper ointments, like **Butt Paste** and **Desitin**, are good moisture barriers.
- Watch for redness and if pressure sores do develop, call a nurse or MD.
- Do not use a plastic or foam donut to relieve pressure.
- Do not massage over bony prominences.

Don't Blame Yourself

Just remember, even with the best care, not all bed sores can be prevented.

HOW TO GIVE A BED BATH

Gather supplies first:

- ❑ waterproof sheet
- ❑ lotion
- ❑ mild soap
- ❑ washcloth and towels
- ❑ wash basin
- ❑ nail brush
- ❑ gloves
- ❑ clean clothes

Before Bath

- Adjust the bed to the right level for you and stand with your feet apart, knees slightly bent and back straight.
- Make sure the room is warm with the door closed to avoid drafts and so the patient doesn't get chilled.
- Offer the bedpan or urinal to the patient before giving the bed bath.
- Wash your hands and put on gloves.
- Remove the patient's clothes and cover him with a light blanket or sheet. Only uncover the area you want to wash.
- Always tell the patient what you're doing even if the person is asleep or unconscious. "I'm going to give you a bath, Charlie. I'm washing your arm now."

Bed Bath

Head

1. Wash from head to toe—starting with the clean and ending with the dirty. Change the water frequently when it becomes cool or dirty.
2. Use one washcloth for soap and one for rinsing. (Cloth should be wet and not dripping.)
3. Start with the face (patient might be able to do this) and use only water for the eyes. Wash with one end of the washcloth and wipe from the center to the outer eye. Then use the other end of the washcloth to do the same with the other eye.
4. Soap washcloth and wash ears, neck, and face. Rinse and pat dry.

Check for Skin Sores

Bathtime is a good time to check for bed sores, rashes, or swelling.

Wash Arms and Hands

1. Place a bath towel under the arm. Wash, rinse, and pat dry. Wash hands and clean under nails with a brush. Then put on deodorant. Repeat with other arm and hand.

Wash Chest

1. Wash the chest. Put towel over the chest and wash, rinse, and dry chest, making sure to wash and dry thoroughly under breasts. Take off towel and pull the sheet up.

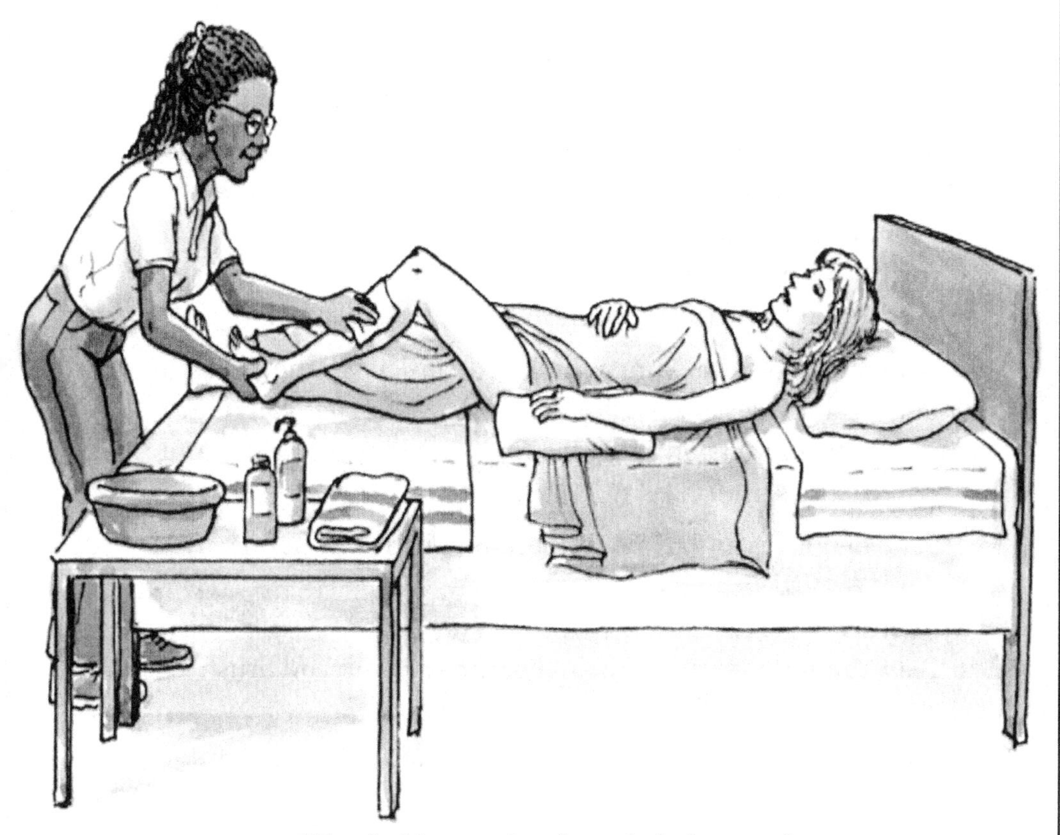

When bathing a patient, leave the body covered except for the part you're washing.

Wash Legs and Feet

1. Remove sheet from one leg, bend the knees, and put a towel under the leg. Wash, rinse, and dry leg and foot. Rub on lotion. (You may want to put the patient's foot in a warm basin to soak.) Do the same with the other leg and foot. Pat dry.
2. Change the water now.
3. Help patient turn on her side and place a towel along her back and bottom. Start at the neck and use long strokes to wash from the neck to the buttocks. Wash, rinse, pat dry, and apply lotion.
4. If you haven't already been wearing gloves, put them on now.
5. Soap up the washcloth and wash the rectal area. Use long strokes down. Rinse and pat dry. Put lotion on her bottom and protective lotions between cheeks, if needed.
6. Change the water and get new washcloth.

Wash Genitals

1. Turn the patient onto her back and wash her genitals.
2. For females, help her to bend her legs, and spread them if she's able. With a soapy washcloth, gently wash the genitals from the front downward, toward the rectum. Rinse after each stroke. Repeat until the area is clean. Pat dry thoroughly with a towel. **Periwash** is an antibacterial cleanser that's good for reducing bacteria in the genital area.
3. For males, if they are uncircumcised, pull down the foreskin and wash, rinse, and pat dry the penis. Make sure you return the foreskin to its original position. Gently wash, rinse and pat dry the scrotum.
4. Take off gloves and dispose of them. Wash your hands.

Final Touches

1. Put a towel under the patient's head, and comb and brush the hair.
2. Help patient into clean bedclothes and make sure he is comfortable.
3. Now is a good time to change the bed linens.

Washing Hair in Bed

Supplies:

- ❑ plastic shampoo tray (or plastic garbage bag)
- ❑ bucket
- ❑ waterproof pad
- ❑ shampoo and conditioner
- ❑ towels
- ❑ pitcher of warm water

Wash Hair

1. If the patient is in hospital bed, adjust the height to a comfortable height for you. (Waist/elbow high)
2. Remember to remove hearing aids, if she has them.
3. Place the waterproof pad under the patient's head and shoulders.
4. Place patient so her head is at the very edge of the bed.
5. Place shampoo tray under her head, and position the drain tube from the tray into the water collection bucket.

Note: If using a plastic bag, place under patient's head and shoulders with a towel on top to soak up excess water. Create a trough by putting rolled up towels under the plastic along sides of the head and under neck. The extra water will roll off the bag into the bucket on the floor.

6. Using the pitcher of warm water, gently pour it over the patient's head.
7. Apply small amount of shampoo and gently massage the scalp.
8. Rinse the hair thoroughly and remove the tray or plastic bag from the bed.
9. Wrap the hair with a large towel. If you want to use a hair dryer, set it on the lowest temperature.

How to Change the Bed Linens

Before: Have clean sheets within reach and a laundry basket for the soiled linens.

1. If patient is in a hospital bed, lower the head and leg sections until the bed is flat. Then raise bed to your elbow level.

2. Remove the head pillow and all covers, except a light top sheet or cotton blanket, to keep the patient warm.
3. If the bed has guardrails, raise the rails on the far side. If not, use a wall or pillows to keep patient secure in the bed.

Begin on the Side Near You

1. Roll the patient onto his side, facing away from you.
2. Roll or fold the top sheet toward the person and tuck it against his back. Now roll or fold the bottom sheet and bed pad against the person's back. Half the bed should now be stripped down to the mattress or mattress pad.

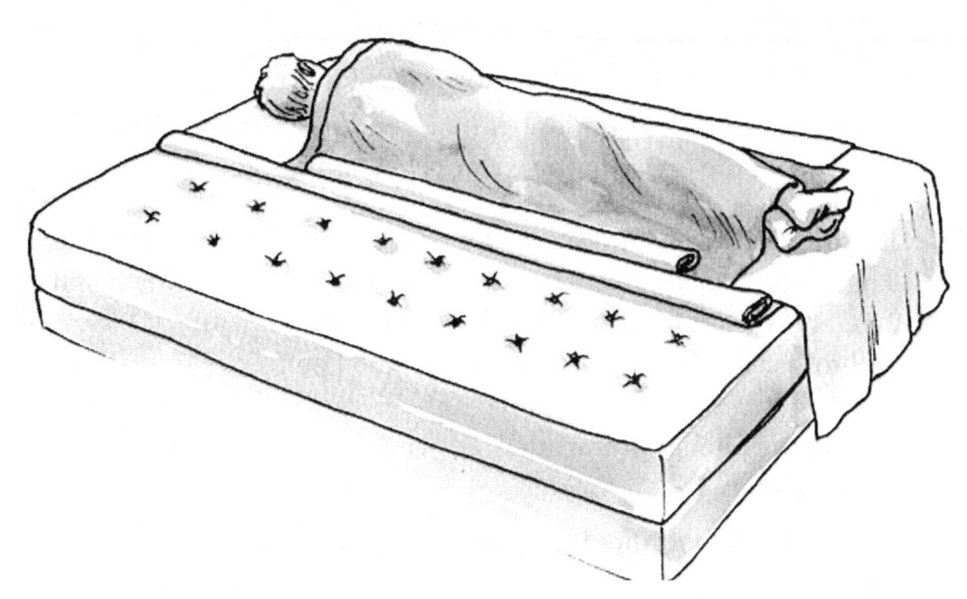

***Basic Theory:** Roll patient to his side, change half the bed, then roll him to the other side, and finish the bed.*

1. **If using a clean flat sheet:** fold it in half, lengthwise, and stretch it against the patient's body from the top to the bottom of the bed.
2. Roll the top half of the clean flat sheet (the half that will go on the other side of the bed) and press it against the patient's body, tucking it under his back.
3. Tuck the remaining portion of the sheet at the head, side and bottom of the bed.

1. **If using a fitted sheet:** Place the fitted corner on the top and bottom corners of the bed nearest you, then smooth the sheet to the center, and tuck it under the patient's back. If you need to add an additional draw sheet, follow the exact same procedure.

Change the Other Side:

1. Roll the patient gently onto his back over the rolled linens that run down the center of the bed and face them toward you. Be sure and raise the guardrail on your side, or stabilize the patient with pillows.
2. Move to the other side of the bed and remove the soiled linens and place them in the laundry basket. This half of the bed should now be stripped down to the mattress or mattress pad.
3. Unroll the clean sheet that's under the patient and pull it tight to make a wrinkle-free bed. Tuck it in at the head, the side and at the foot of the bed. Pull any additional pads or draw sheet away from and center and tuck anything that might hang over the side of the bed under the mattress.
4. Change the pillow case.
5. Roll the patient onto his back and change the top sheet.
6. When you tuck in the top sheet at the bottom of the bed, be sure to leave room for the patient to move his feet comfortably.
7. Spread a blanket over the top sheet—too heavy a blanket can cause discomfort and pain. If this is a problem, use a blanket support that sits under the blankets and raises the blanket off the patient's body.
8. Position the patient so he is comfortable.

NINE

SYMPTOM MANAGEMENT

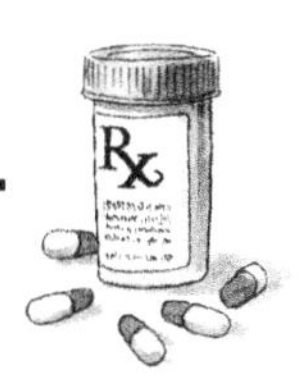

WHAT TO DO WHEN THINGS GO WRONG

Don't panic. Every day is a new day in caregiving and things can change fast. Problems can range from a tiny bedsore to severe nausea and vomiting. Some symptoms are easy to take care of, while others are more challenging. Either way, don't hit the panic button. There's almost always something you can do to make your loved one more comfortable.

Never Hesitate To Call Your Healthcare Provider

The goal is to keep your loved one clean, comfortable and pain free. If you don't know what to do about a symptom, call for advice.

When to Call 911 or Go to the Emergency Room

Most dying people don't want to go to the ER They prefer to stay in their homes. If the patient is on hospice, call the hospice nurse first to be sure you need an ER visit. Reasons to go to the emergency room:

- A broken bone or fractured hip.
- Any distressing symptoms that cannot be managed at home, like an uncontrollable nosebleed or a cut that needs stitches.
- In rare instances, a patient on hospice may need to go into the hospital if his symptoms (like severe pain) cannot be controlled at home.

Symptoms and Solutions by page number

The following pages are an alphabetical listing of some common problems, their probable causes, and what you can do to help.

Achiness 95
Anxiety / Agitation 95
Bedsores or Pressure Injuries 97
Bladder Spasms 98
Bleeding 98
Breathing Difficulties 100
Combativeness. 101
Confusion 102
Constipation 104
Dementia at the End of Life 106
Diarrhea / Cramps 107
Dry Mouth and Thirst. 108
Fever. 108
Hallucinations 109
Hiccups 110
Incontinence 111
Insomnia 112
Itching 113
Jaundice 115
Mouth Sores 115
Nausea / Vomiting 116
Rash 117
Seizures 118
Sudden Severe Pain 119
Swallowing Difficulties / Throat Secretions 120
Swelling 120
Urination Painful / Difficult 122

SYMPTOMS

When you see this image, a doctor or nurse must first be consulted before administering any of the prescription medicines mentioned in this chapter. Your doctor should also know any other medications and over-the-counter meds, like Advil and Tylenol or supplements, the patient is taking.

ACHINESS: GENERAL END-OF-LIFE ACHINESS

Causes:

- Chronic problems like arthritis or old injuries—joints, muscles, bones
- Inactivity and being in one position too long can result in decreased circulation
- General aches in the muscles and joints can happen as the body shuts down, especially in the last few days.

What can I do for achiness?

1. Heating pads, ice, passive exercises in bed (Lifting the arm or leg, bending the elbow or knee), massaging the legs and arms, and turning patients in bed

2. Put a foam or egg crate pad on top of the mattress to make the bed more comfortable.

3. Try **Tylenol** or other non-prescription pain relievers like **Advil** or **Aleve.**

Medications for achiness:

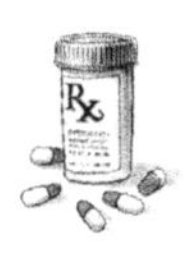

- Toward the end of life, physicians often prescribe small drops of **morphine** in the cheek.

ANXIETY AND AGITATION

Anxiety can trigger extreme restlessness and an inability to relax or sleep. A patient may have difficulty breathing or may be unable to concentrate on anything but her fears. As she becomes more agitated she may raise her voice or strike out.

Causes (Anxiety and Agitation Continued):

- Stress, fear, and worrying about dying
- Difficulty breathing
- Brain tumors and liver disease
- New medications
- Dementia
- Pain
- Full bladder
- Constipation
- Infection

What can I do for anxiety and agitation?

1. Rule out problems that can be solved: the patient could have a full bladder or be feeling pain somewhere, which is making her anxious. Then address the problem: take her to the bathroom, or find out what is hurting and give pain medications, or address breathing difficulties with meds.
2. If anxiety is from fear, ask the patient to talk about her feelings. Often times just talking about fears can help alleviate the anxiety. Include an outside counselor if needed.
3. For general anxiety, ask the patient to do deep breathing, which will calm the body. Instruct your patient to take slow, deep breaths in through her nose and out, with pursed lips (like blowing up a balloon).
4. Try using distraction with music, watching movies, or going for a walk or drive.
5. Use relaxation techniques such as visualization and massage.

Medication for Anxiety and Agitation:

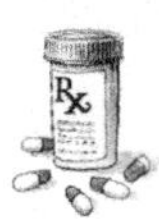

- For general anxiety: doctors often prescribe medications like **Ativan, Xanax,** and **Valium.**
- For severe agitation, especially for a patient with dementia, and those having delusions and hallucinations: **Haldol** and **Seroquel** are often prescribed.
- If the patient is having disease–related shortness of breath, doctors would recommend **morphine.**

BEDSORES OR PRESSURE INJURIES

Prevention is the key!

Bedsores or pressure injuries develop when an area of the skin has decreased blood supply, so nutrients and oxygen can't get to it. The most susceptible spots are the areas where the skin is close to the bone: back of the head, ears, shoulder bones, spine, elbows, tailbone, hip bones, heels, and ankles.

Causes of bedsores or pressure sores:

- When the patient lies in one position too long, sores develop at the pressure points.
- Sitting in a chair or wheelchair for too long, without moving.
- Poor nutrition and dehydration can make a patient more susceptible to skin breakdown.
- Lying in urine and feces for too long
- Sores can appear when a patient isn't bathed enough or when the skin and the vulnerable bony areas stay moist.
- Pressure sores can result from the friction of the patient's skin against the sheet when he is moved in the bed. It's called a "shear" or "sheet burn."

What can I do for bedsores?

1. Keep the patient off the sores and reddened areas as much as you can. Change the patient's position: if she is still active, encourage her to move around. If she is bedbound or chairbound, try to turn or change her position every 2 to 4 hours.
2. Never attempt to treat a pressure sore yourself. You need to consult a healthcare professional. They have special training in treating ulcers.
3. It's never too late to put air mattresses or foam pads on the bed.
4. It's really important to know that not all skin breakdown and pressure sores can be avoided.

To treat the bedsore's odor: Sprinkle **Flagyl** powder (prescription needed) on the wound tissue. Put a pan of kitty litter under the bed.

Katie

Toward the end, my Dad was developing sores on his coccyx, but he wasn't able to lie on his side because of his breathing problems. I rolled him on to his side and we put a little pillow under his back above the sore, and another below the sore creating a pocket of air, so that his back wasn't touching the bed when I rolled him back.

BLADDER SPASMS

Spasms feel like a sudden cramping and are often painful.

Causes:

- Urinary tract infections
- Tumors in the bladder
- Nerve damage from diseases (Parkinson's, diabetes, MS)
- The insertion of a catheter may cause a feeling that makes a patient feel like he constantly has to go to the bathroom

Note: Spasms may cause leaking around the catheter, even if there is urine in the tubing.

What can I do for bladder spasms?

1. A heating pad or hot water bottle on the abdomen relaxes the bladder.

Medications for Bladder Spasms:

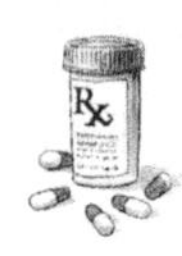

- Urinary tract infections are treated with antibiotics. Doctors often prescribe **Pyridium** to relieve pain until antibiotics kick in. (Pyridium turns urine dark red or orange. Don't be alarmed.)
- Catheter cramping usually goes away the next day, but **Ditropan** can help relax the bladder.

BLEEDING

Bleeding is rare and, most of the time, not painful. But it can be distressing.

Causes:

- Blood thinners (**Coumadin, Lovenox,** too much **Advil**)
- Diseases, like liver disease and leukemia, that cause clotting disorders
- Liver disease can cause swollen veins in the esophagus to rupture.
- Lung cancer may occasionally cause coughing up of blood.
- Esophageal and throat cancer may cause spitting up of blood.
- Uterine and cervical cancer can cause vaginal bleeding. Urinary tract cancers (kidney, bladder) can cause blood in urine.
- GI tract cancers (mouth, esophagus, stomach, colon, bowel, rectum) can cause bleeding out of the mouth or blood in the stool, which looks dark or black, and sticky or tarry.

What can I do for bleeding?

1. Remain calm. Bleeding is probably not painful for the patient.
2. Call your healthcare provider if the patient is on blood thinners. The dose might need to be adjusted.
3. If a patient starts vomiting blood, it is usually more distressing for the family than the patient. If she is in bed, turn her on her side and use dark towels to clean up the blood. Then call your healthcare provider.
4. If bleeding is excessive, and you're scared, call the doctor. If you are on hospice, call the hospice nurse.

Medications for Bleeding:

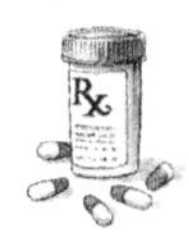

- If the symptoms include anxiety, nausea, or pain, medications are available: **Ativan** is generally prescribed for anxiety; **Zofran** or **Compazine** for nausea; and **morphine** for pain.
- For severe esophageal bleeding, the esophagus can be banded by a doctor.
- If the patient is having symptoms of anemia (weakness, shortness of breath and extreme fatigue), a blood transfusion might be ordered if appropriate.
- **Versed** nasal spray or **Thorazine** suppositories for sedation if needed.

Nosebleeds

Nosebleeds are caused by: blood thinners, diseases that cause clotting disorders, dry air, tumors in the nose, blowing the nose a lot, and plain old nose picking. Here's what you can do for nose bleeds:

1. Have patient sit up and lean forward so the blood flows out, rather than back into the throat.
2. Pinch nose on the soft part of the nose (breathe through the mouth) and hold for 5 minutes. If still bleeding, hold for another 5 minutes.
3. Put an icepack to the back of the neck or on the upper chest.
4. Sometimes a squirt of the decongestant nasal spray, **Afrin**, will stop it.
5. If it persists, call the nurse or healthcare provider. (Occasionally patients will go to the hospital to have the nose cauterized.)

BREATHING DIFFICULTIES

Breathing distress (also called dyspnea and air hunger) is very common at the end of life and can cause anxiety and panic in the patient. Signs to look for are: rapid breathing, use of the muscles in the neck and chest to gasp for air, bluish color to lips and fingertips, and gasping, wheezing, and grunting.

Causes:

- Lung congestion
- Tumor spread
- Anemia
- Abdominal distention from enlarged organs or tumors
- Heart failure
- Anxiety
- Airway constriction from emphysema, asthma, COPD or other reactive airway diseases
- Extra fluid in the space around the lungs
- Increased airway secretions

What can I do for breathing difficulties?

1. Keep calm. Raise the head of the patient's bed.
2. A fan in the room relieves shortness of breath by moving the air.
3. If the patient has copious secretions and is choking, turn him way over on his side, even hanging his head off the bed, to drain out the mucous. Gently pound on back.
4. You can even use a washcloth to remove the secretions.

Medications for Breathing Difficulties:

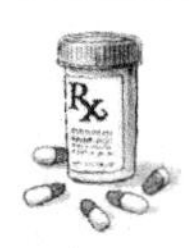

- **Morphine** and other narcotics like **Dilaudid** and **oxycodone** are the best medications for disease-related breathing difficulties.
- **Ativan** will help anxiety.
- **Furosemide** is sometimes prescribed for lung congestion—it is a diuretic that removes extra fluid from the inside of the lungs.
- Inhalers or nebulizing treatments
- **Thorazine** can be prescribed for extreme, persistent air hunger, and for sedation of the patient, near the end of life
- If the fluid is around the lung, a doctor can tap the space to drain the fluid out (thoracentesis).
- For thick secretions, use **Mucinex** or **guaifenesin syrup**.
- Medications to dry up secretions: **Robinul, atropine** drops in mouth, **scopolamine** patch.

Why Morphine Helps with Shortness of Breath

Morphine relaxes the blood vessels, so the heart doesn't have to work so hard. With the heart not working as hard and needing less oxygen, it stops sending distress signals to the brain. It slows and makes each breath more effective. It also helps deaden some of the natural chemical substances in your body that cause you to become tense and excited.

COMBATIVENESS

Extreme agitation that results in the patient refusing care and even striking out and yelling at caregivers is distressing. The more upset the patient gets, the calmer you need to be.

Causes:

- Alzheimer's and other dementias
- Brain tumors
- Liver disease can cause extreme agitation, which could lead to combativeness.
- Infection
- Extreme pain
- Full bladder or bowel impactions (especially in people with dementia)
- New medications
- Lack of oxygen to the brain from different lung diseases

What can I do for combativeness?

1. Talk calmly and slowly to the patient. Don't argue with him.
2. Try distraction, such as calm music, singing, or sitting and talking.
3. For your own safety, don't force care on the patient without help.
4. If you suspect a urinary tract infection, call your doctor or nurse about an antibiotic.
5. Address possible other problems like full bladder or pain that might be causing the combativeness.

Medications for Combativeness:

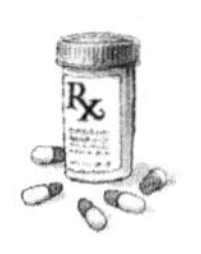

- **Haldol** in pill, liquid or gel (rub on the wrist).
- If the patient can't swallow medications, doctors often prescribe **Thorazine** suppositories (after the patient is calmed down).
- Some patients have to be kept sedated to be able to provide care safely. Or if they're out of control, they may require a 24-hour care facility.

Jahnna
Dad would go through bouts of combativeness where he wouldn't let me into his room, or he'd suddenly decide he had to go somewhere and couldn't be talked out of it. I found if I sang my responses to him, either in a familiar tune or just a playful way, he'd come around. When we needed him to walk, I'd sing, "You put your right foot in, you put your right foot out. Then you grab your walker and shake it all about." He'd suddenly start doing a little funny wiggle with his bottom. The conga was also a good method of getting him aimed in the right direction. I'd hold onto his waist and dance the conga where we were headed. Singing really was the key in our household for getting him to do something, or to get him out of an awful mood.

CONFUSION

Confusion can be present in patients, especially during the dying process.

Causes:

- Medications, especially narcotics and tranquilizers
- Lack of oxygen to the brain—generally from lung cancer or COPD
- Kidney failure causing a build-up of waste products in the blood.
- Liver failure causing a build-up of ammonia in the blood
- High blood calcium from cancer
- Infection
- Pain
- A full bladder can cause restlessness and agitation.
- Dementia and Alzheimer's
- Organ Failure is a normal part of the dying process. As the organs shut down, they can no longer circulate blood through the body and clear toxins from the blood. Confusion and restlessness may be a result.

Sundowning

It's common for people with dementia to get more confused and agitated as the sun goes down. There is no known cause for it, but as the light disappears and it becomes dark out they can become really disruptive. It may be that this is the point in the day when they are finally really exhausted, like little kids around dinner time. Or it may actually have to do with a fear of the dark or the shadows that appear. Try turning the lights on in the early afternoon, to make the transition through "the witching hour" easier. Try medicating before the agitation begins.

Sudden Changes in Behavior

If one day an elderly patient is able to dress and feed herself, and the next day she's combative, confused, and even incontinent–a urinary tract or bladder infection is the likely culprit. Many elderly patients' falls are actually a result of their reaction to a urinary tract infection. They suffer pain and confusion, and have that sudden urge to race to the bathroom, and then fall. Have a urine sample tested. Antibiotics may be prescribed.

What can I do for confusion?

1. If there is an abrupt onset of confusion, check to see if any new medications have been started, and contact your nurse or MD to see about stopping them.
2. If pain is the cause, ask the patient where he hurts.
3. Look for signs, like moaning or grunting, clutching a part of the body, grimacing, or holding stiff and trying not to move. Give pain meds as per plan. If it's a new pain, call your healthcare provider.
4. Check patient to see if she has been urinating regularly. A catheter may be needed if she is having urinary retention.
5. If the patient has a catheter, make sure it's in full working order.

Medications for Confusion:

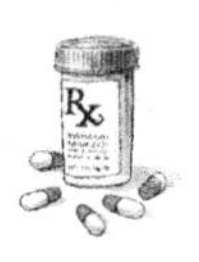

- If low oxygen level is suspected, the nurse or healthcare provider can check it and order oxygen to be delivered. If the patient is close to death, oxygen is not recommended, but comfort meds can be used to relieve symptoms.
- If there is high ammonia in the blood from liver failure, doctors prescribe **Lactulose** to pull the ammonia out of the blood stream and into the intestines.
- If all other causes have been ruled out, physicians often treat restlessness with **Ativan, Xanax,** and **Haldol**; and agitation with **Haldol, Depakote,** and **Seroquel.**

Helping Your Confused Loved One

- Don't argue with the patient about what she is experiencing or thinking.
- Keep a nightlight on because patients may not know where they are in the dark.
- Keep a clock visible that shows the time and day of the week.
- Post photographs by the bed.
- Keep doors closed except to rooms that you want the patient to have access to, like the bathroom or bedroom.
- Have someone, besides a family member, sit with the patient–like an old friend or chaplain. This can provide a calming presence.

CONSTIPATION

The patient should have at least one bowel movement every three days—ideally more often. Even if a person is no longer eating, the body still produces about ¼ cup of stool a day.

Causes:

- Drugs
- Inactivity
- Dehydration and decreased diet
- Tumor growth

Narcotics Cause Constipation!

Every patient on pain medicine should have a bowel plan in place. If they don't have a plan, most people will get constipated! The best treatment for constipation? Prevention.

Untreated Constipation Can Lead to a Stool Impaction, which is very hard stool in the lower bowel. This can be very painful with liquid stool sometimes leaking around the hard mass. Do not give an enema. This may require a manual disimpaction by a health care professional or a trip to the ER if patient isn't on hospice.

What can I do for constipation?

1. Bowel stimulants almost always need to be taken when a patient is on narcotics. **Senakot** is a combination of stool softener and stimulant.

2. **Ducolax, Miralax, Lactulose,** or **Milk of Magnesia** can be taken alone, mixed in with a little prune juice, or stirred into tea.
3. **Smooth Move Tea** (once a day)
4. Prunes or prune juice or a simple warm liquid, like coffee or tea, can help.
5. Increase fluids, as tolerated and include daily physical activity if possible.
6. Swallowing a couple of tablespoons of mineral oil can soften the stool. Olive oil with a little lemon juice also works.
7. A very warm washcloth pressed against the anus can help a patient struggling to have a bowel movement.

Note: **Metamucil** is not generally recommended unless the patient is taking in lots of fluids. Otherwise, it may have the opposite affect and bind him up.

How to Give an Enema

Pre-caution: check with nurse or MD before giving an enema to a patient with heart disease, severe abdominal pain, a bleeding disorder, rectal bleeding, or hard stool in the rectum.

Supplies: gloves, lubricant (**KY gel**), and a pre-packaged enema (**Fleets**) or an enema bag filled with 1 to 2 quarts warm water, and a little baking soda or salt.

1. Patient should be lying on her left side with legs bent, with a waterproof pad or towel underneath her.
2. Apply lubricant to the applicator. Also put lubricant on the anus. If using enema bag, run solution through the tube to clear air from the bag.
3. Slowly insert the applicator at an angle toward the small of the back, about 3 inches or until you meet resistance.
4. Enema bag should be 12 to 18 inches above the body. Slowly release the liquid. If the patient cramps—stop and wait till the cramp is gone.
5. **Fleets:** Slowly squeeze the bottle until it's empty.
6. Instruct the patient to hold the liquid in as long as she can (usually 5 to 10 minutes).
7. Help her to the commode or toilet.

Dementia at the End of Life

Dementia is a general term for a decline in mental ability as marked by memory loss, paranoia, personality changes, and impaired reasoning. It is a disease and not a symptom, but many elderly patients suffer from dementia. Alzheimer's is the most common form.

Causes:

Physical changes to the brain cells by disease or injury. While most dementia is permanent and worsens over time, some confusion and memory loss can be caused by:

- Depression
- Medication side effects
- Excess use of alcohol
- A UTI (urinary tract infection)
- Thyroid problems
- Vitamin deficiencies
- Dehydration

Symptoms:

- Memory loss
- Confusion
- Impaired reasoning
- Confusion with time and place
- Changes in mood and personality
- Becoming suspicious, afraid, angry, and sometimes striking out

What can I do?

1. Caring for a loved one who is dying is hard enough, but when your loved one has dementia, it is frustrating and heartbreaking. Stay calm. Speak in a reassuring voice, and eliminate distractions, like TV.
2. Keep communication simple: don't over-explain. Don't argue.
3. If she is suddenly angry or upset, it may be that she is in pain but can't really identify it. Taking an **aspirin, Tylenol,** or **Advil** might calm her down.
4. Remember kicking, biting and hitting is often fueled by fear or helplessness. Don't argue. Try distracting her. If nothing works, give her space and a chance to reset.
5. Try to stay pleasant and reassuring. Compliment her on accomplishing simple tasks. "Good job."
6. Try activities like reading to patient, music, pet therapy, and reminiscing by looking through old photos and magazines

Medications for the Symptoms of Dementia

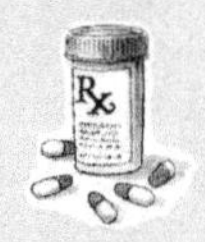

- **Ativan** or **Xanax** is used for anxiety. Use cautiously, because they may have the opposite effect.
- **Haldol** and **Seroquel** is used for agitation.

DIARRHEA AND CRAMPS

Diarrhea is loose or watery stools passed 3 or 4 times a day.

Causes:

- Infection
- Food sensitivity
- Anxiety
- Medication
- GI infection (C. diff)
- Disorders (like short bowel) or injuries of the intestinal tract
- A bowel impaction

What can I do for diarrhea and cramps?

1. **Imodium** is sold over the counter and will control diarrhea. Call doctor or nurse first.
2. Use the BRAT diet: bananas, white rice, applesauce, and bananas.
3. Offer clear liquids and tea.
4. Avoid fresh fruits and vegetables.
5. Avoid very hot and very cold drinks—they stimulate the bowels.
6. Avoid caffeinated beverages.
7. If the condition continues for more than a couple of days, call your healthcare provider.
8. Be sure that the patient is cleaned well after each bowel movement. You may also want to apply a soothing cream or moisture barrier to the anal area, especially if the patient is incontinent.

Medications for Diarrhea and Cramps:

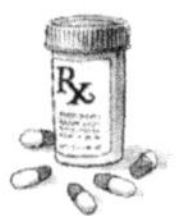

- If infection is the causing the diarrhea the doctor may prescribe an antibiotic.

Note: If the patient has not had regular bowel movements for several days, but has very loose stools leaking out of the rectum, this can actually be a sign of a bowel impaction. You would not want to treat this problem with **Imodium**! Call your healthcare provider.

Dry Mouth and Thirst

Dry mouth is a very common problem where the mouth produces little or no saliva. People with dry mouth have trouble eating, swallowing, talking and wearing dentures.

Causes

- Medications
- Mouth breathing
- Oxygen
- General dehydration

What can I do?

1. Offer lozenges and sour lemon drops for the patient to suck on.
2. Add ¼ tsp of **glycerine** to 1 cup of water. Swish and spit—don't swallow. It acts as a moisturizer.
3. Avoid foods that really need to be chewed.
4. Moisten foods with yogurt, sauces, and gravy.
5. Ice chips, frozen popsicles, frozen grapes, and watermelon are easy to eat.
6. Use an over the counter artificial saliva spray, swab, or solution such as **Salivart.** Coconut oil also works.
7. Have patient sleep with a humidifier.
8. Add humidity to the oxygen supply.
9. Keep a water bottle nearby.
10. Use a moisturizer on lips, because they dry up too.
11. **Biotene** makes special dry mouth toothpastes and chewing gum.

FEVER

It is common for a patient's body temperature to spike as she nears death.

Causes

- The body's inability to regulate temperature as the organs shut down
- Infection

What can I do for a fever?

1. If the fever is causing discomfort, offer **Tylenol.** If the patient can't swallow, you can use Tylenol suppositories.
2. Strip the patient and cover with a light sheet.
3. Give a sponge bath with lukewarm water.
4. Put cool washcloths on the forehead.

Medications for Fevers:

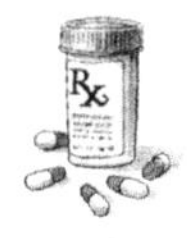

- If infection is causing the fever, a doctor may prescribe antibiotics.

Jahnna
I didn't realize that Dad was having a high fever. He had been breathing quickly and didn't appear to be sweating. But I discovered his pillow was soaked. I quickly put a cool washcloth on his head and his breathing seemed to slow.

HALLUCINATIONS

Patients often have hallucinations, or visions, as they approach death in the last weeks to days. It's not unusual for people close to death to see friends or relatives who have died, standing in the room with them. Many people see their mothers and call out to them. Some people see angels or Jesus at their bedside. Sometimes patients have conversations with their visions—listening and responding.

Causes for Hallucinations:

- Medications
- Toxins in the blood
- Low oxygen
- Electrolyte imbalance
- The mystery of death

End of Life Visions

Marcus was a young fireman who had barely been married a year. Three days before he died, Marcus was lying in bed with his wife curled up against him. He had been dozing in and out. Suddenly he opened his eyes and smiled. He gestured to the whole (empty) room and said, "Everybody! I want you to meet my wife Emily." Emily cried with happiness. She felt that her young husband would not be alone on his journey into the unknown.

What can I do for hallucinations?

1. Don't feel you need to argue with or correct the patient.
2. You may want to ask about the "visions" and have the patient describe them to you.

Medications for Hallucinations:

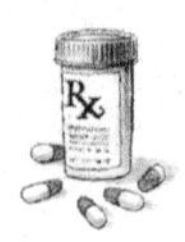

- If the hallucinations are disturbing and cause the patient to be agitated, your healthcare provider may prescribe medications like **Haldol** or **Seroquel.**

HICCUPS

It's not unusual for a dying patient to have a case of the hiccups. Hiccups are irritable spasms of the diaphragm muscle.

Causes:

- Abdominal bloating
- Electrolyte imbalance or the build-up in the blood of harmful substances
- Kidney and liver failure
- Strokes
- Brain tumors
- Esophageal, stomach, and lung cancer
- Stress, anxiety
- Drinking very hot or very cold or carbonated drinks
- Irritation of the nerves that stretch from the neck to the chest

What can I do for hiccups?

1. Drink a cup of water with a teaspoon of vinegar in it.
2. Have the patient rebreathe into a paper bag—increased carbon dioxide in the blood can stop hiccups.
3. Or try to do this as quickly as possible:

Step 1: Inhale as much air into your lungs as you can.

Step 2: Swallow but don't let any air out.

Step 3: Inhale some more. It may not be a lot, but do the best you can.

Step 4: Swallow again. Don't let any air out!

Step 5: Inhale some more and then swallow. Your lungs should be achingly full.

Step 6: Exhale.

Medications for Hiccups:

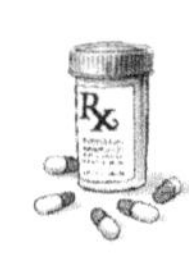

- For severe hiccups: **Thorazine, Reglan,** or **Baclofen** might be prescribed.

INCONTINENCE

The inability to control the bladder or bowels.

Causes:

- As patients reach the end of life, muscles weaken and they may not feel the urge to go.
- Urinary tract infection (The urine can have a strong, foul odor.)
- Anti-depressant medications and diuretics
- Prostate and bladder cancer
- Constipation (An impacted bowel can press on bladder.)
- Neuromuscular diseases: ALS, MS, and spinal cord tumors and injuries
- Enlarged prostate
- Dementia

What can I do for incontinence?

- Eliminate the cause, such as infection or medications, if possible.
- Bedpan or bedside commode (Set a schedule and offer every 2 hours while patient is awake to prevent accidents.)
- Briefs (Pull-ups for adults) or adult diapers
- Pads which can be inserted into the briefs
- Waterproof/absorbent pads for chairs and beds
- Waterproof mattress pads to go under the sheets
- Urinal—portable pitcher that can be kept by the bed or chair

Medications for Incontinence:

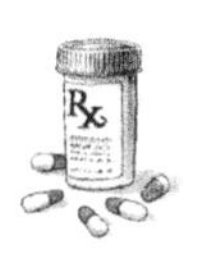

- **Flomax** can help reduce the frequent urge to go in male patients.
- **Ditropan** may help with urge incontinence.
- **Antibiotic** if an infection is present

Using a Catheter

The condom catheter is for men. It slips over the penis and is secured to it with double-sided tape (the area should be shaved to avoid pulling hair).

The in-dwelling catheter for women and men is a small tube inserted into the bladder that continually drains urine into a bag.

Catheter Alert

When a catheter is inserted in an un-circumcised male, make sure the foreskin is pulled back up after the catheter is inserted. If it is not, the penis can become very swollen and painful.

INSOMNIA

Patients at the end of life often experience difficulty falling asleep or staying asleep.

Causes:

- Insomnia can be caused by physical problems and emotional worries.
- Some patients are afraid to go to sleep for fear of not waking up.
- Medications, like **Decadron**, can rev patients up and keep them awake.
- Lying back on the bed causes breathing problems and keeps them awake
- Patients report that they "Just can't turn their mind off," worrying about what's going to happen to them, their family, their business, etc.
- Some patients get their days and nights mixed up, sleeping in the daytime, and then being wide awake at night.
- Pain may be worse at night when the patient has fewer distractions.

What can I do for insomnia?

1. The first thing to do is to set up a regular bedtime routine for the patient: put on pajamas, brush teeth, take meds, go to bed.

2. Offer a glass of warm milk, **Sleepy Time Tea,** or wine.
3. Turn off the TV. Television just before bed can keep the mind racing, especially with demented patients.
4. Massage
5. Play soft music before bedtime. Harp music induces tone-generated gamma waves that help you relax.
6. Patients who are afraid to go to sleep appreciate you sitting quietly by their bedside until they go to sleep.
7. If breathing is a problem, it may help the patient to have oxygen at night.
8. Raise the head of the bed to make breathing easier.
9. Leave an extra dose of pain medication by the bedside with a glass of water, in case the patient wakes up in pain.

Medications for insomnia:

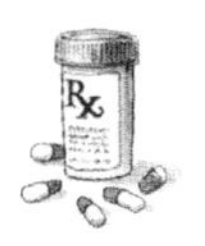

- Some antidepressants help with sleep.
- **Xanax** and **Ativan** can help with anxiety and worry, if that is the problem.
- Medications like **morphine** or **Ativan** are often prescribed to help with breathing problems.
- If the patient isn't sleeping because of agitation, doctors might prescribe **Haldol** or **Seroquel** to calm him.
- If the patient wakes up because of pain, give additional pain medication at bedtime. Pain meds can range from **ibuprofen** to **Vicoden** to **morphine.** Ask your healthcare provider about a time-released pain pill at night.
- If all else fails, your healthcare provider can prescribe a sleeping pill like **Trazadone** or **Remeron.**

ITCHING

Most of the time itching affects the arms, legs, and torso, but it can be anywhere on the body.

ITCHING (continued)

Causes :

- Reactions to medications
- Kidney failure
- Jaundice from liver failure
- Dry skin
- Yeast infections
- Peripheral neuropathy—usually on feet or hands—from chemotherapy or diabetes
- Cancer treatments
- Cancer: Hodgkin's lymphoma, pancreatic cancer, leukemia, Kaposi's sarcoma, AIDs, liver metastases, breast cancer, prostate cancer, and brain tumors can cause all over itching.
- Toxins in the blood

What can I do for itching?

1. Avoid hot water and bathing excessively. Use soap sparingly.
2. Keep the room temperature cool.
3. Have patient wear loose cotton clothing.
4. Use lubricating lotions containing oil that moistens dry skin.
5. Try anti-itch lotions: **Aveeno, Sarna** and **hydrocortisone** creams (a stronger hydrocortisone cream can be prescribed by a doctor).
6. Use an electric shaver instead of a razor.
7. Put an ice pack on the area.
8. Pinch or pat area instead of scratching.
9. Offer over-the-counter antihistamine medication, like **Benadryl.**
10. Distract the patient with music, guided imagery, and foot rubs.

Medications for Itching:

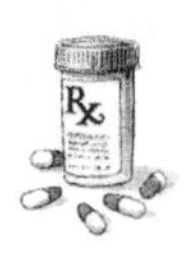

- **Atarax** or **Vistaril** for allergic reactions
- Some types of antidepressant medicines like **Elavil, Tophranil,** and **Paxil** work well for itching due to nerve irritation, such as peripheral neuropathy.
- **Prednisone** is often prescribed for severe allergic skin reactions.
- **Zofran,** which is an anti-nausea drug, can be effective in treating itching caused by liver disease, and the use of opiates, like morphine.
- **Diflucan** is an antifungal that treats yeast infections.

JAUNDICE

A yellow color of the skin, eyes, or mucous membranes. The yellow color comes from bilirubin, which is a by-product of old, red blood cells. Bilirubin is what gives stools their brownish color. Patients with jaundice can have pale or clay-colored stools. Urine may become dark.

Causes:

- Cancers such as liver, pancreatic, and gall bladder
- Hepatitis
- Liver failure
- Side effect of radiation or chemo-therapy

What can I do for jaundice?

There is nothing you can do to stop the jaundice. It's not painful. This is just an inevitable side effect of certain diseases.

MOUTH SORES

Mouth sores are like having cuts or ulcers in the mouth. They may be very red, or have small white patches in the middle (candida thrush), and they may bleed.

Causes:

- Sores are common after chemotherapy.
- Oxygen therapy
- Steroid inhalers and pills
- Dehydration
- Infection
- Poor mouth care
- Lack of protein

What can I do for mouth sores?

1. The key to healing or avoiding mouth sores is to clean the mouth twice a day.
2. Gently rinse the mouth with 1 tsp of baking soda and 1 cup of warm water after meals and at bedtime. This can help with pain relief.
3. If using an inhaler, rinse with water or a baking soda solution immediately afterwards. Avoid mouthwashes that contain salt, alcohol, or other irritants.
4. Gently brush the teeth with a soft toothbrush. Soak the bristles in hot water to soften them.

What can I do for mouth sores? (Continued)

5. If brushing hurts too much, patient can use a toothette, which is a small sponge on a stick. If the patient has ulcers, don't use the toothette; use cotton swabs dipped in cold water.
6. Ice chips or frozen fruit popsicles can provide some relief.
7. Keep the mouth moist with a spray bottle with a few drops of vegetable oil in the water.
8. If the patient wears dentures and has severe mouth sores, take the dentures out to let the mouth rest. (At least at night.)

Medications for Mouth Sores:

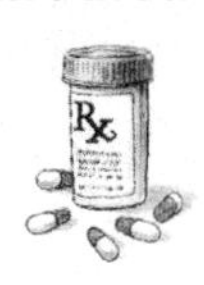

- "**Miracle Mouthwash**"—a pharmacist mixes equal parts of **Maalox, Benadryl,** and viscous **Lidocaine.** Swish with this pain reliever before meals, at bedtime, and as needed.
- **Nystatin** or **Diflucan** for yeast in mouth.

NAUSEA AND VOMITING

Causes:

- Drugs
- Chemotherapy
- Anxiety
- Cancer tumors
- Stomach flu
- Strong tastes or smells
- Increased pressure in the head, which can be from brain tumors or strokes
- Bowel obstruction

What can I do for nausea and vomiting?

1. Administer nausea or pain medications an hour before eating.
2. Ginger tea or peppermint tea can soothe the stomach.
3. Avoid strong cooking odors or perfumes.
4. Serve food cold or at room temperature to decrease its smell and taste.
5. Offer small sips of carbonated soda, like ginger ale, Coca Cola, Seven-Up—let the beverage sit for a short time before offering.
6. Patient should not lie flat for at least an hour after eating.

7. The BRAT diet—bananas, rice, applesauce, and toast—allows the GI tract to rest. Saltines or toast are also foods they can usually swallow.
8. Offer cool, clear beverages such as broth, apple juice, and tea.

Medications for Nausea:

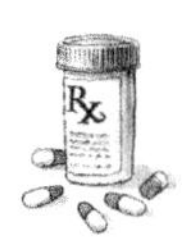

- **Zofran, Compazine** (which also comes in a suppository), and **Reglan** are anti-nausea medications.
- **Ativan,** which is an anti-anxiety medication, helps nausea.
- **Haldol,** in small amounts, can really help with nausea.
- **Decadron** is a steroid that may help.

Bowel Obstruction

If a bowel obstruction is causing the nausea and vomiting, contact the health-care provider immediately. Signs are: distended abdomen, inability to have a bowel movement, severe vomiting–sometimes of fecal matter. The patient should not eat or drink anything at this point, but small sips of water or ice chips are probably okay.

If pain and nausea symptoms are severe and can't be controlled by other means, comfort medications can be administered in suppository form or by pump.

RASH

Rashes can easily develop in a sedentary patient. They usually appear in the warm, moist areas of the body.

Causes:

- Yeast infections are the most common cause. The rash looks like little red dots and appears in the groin/buttocks area, and under the breasts.
- Diaper rash is a result of constant wetness from incontinence.
- Adverse reaction to a new medication can cause a rash.

What can I do for rashes?

1. Keep area around the scrotum and the breasts dry.

What can I do for rashes? (Continued)

2. For diaper rash, apply a skin barrier like **Butt Paste** or **Desitin.** Change diaper frequently. If the rash continues, consider a catheter.
3. For a yeast rash: Rub into the skin folds and diaper area an antifungal moisture barrier or powder, like **Zeasorb. Miconazole** is an anti-fungal agent that is in a lot of over-the-counter creams.
4. Call nurse if new medication was just started. It might be the cause.
5. See Itching (pg. 113–114) if it happens with rash.

Medications for Rashes:

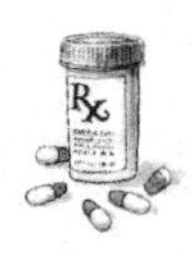

- **Miconazole, Diflucan,** or **Nystatin** are good for yeast infections.
- **Prednisone** for severe allergic rashes

SEIZURES

Seizures are rare. They are sudden involuntary convulsive movements of the muscles. Jerky, uncoordinated movements, headache, blurred vision, sweating, stomach-ache, or breathing difficulties may all be signs that a seizure is about to happen. It usually lasts less than 5 minutes, and the patient may lose control of her bladder. It can leave the patient exhausted and confused for several hours.

Causes:

- Brain tumors
- Cancers, like lung, breast, or melanoma that have spread to the brain
- Metabolic problems
- Anemia
- Chemotherapy drugs or radiation
- Strokes
- Sudden withdrawal of certain meds and alcohol

What can I do for seizures?

1. During the seizure: lay the patient down if you can. Turn her on her side in case she vomits. Keep her from hurting herself by padding with pillows.
2. Do not put anything between her teeth—you could injure the teeth or jaw.

Medications for Seizures:

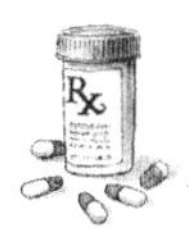

- **Valium**, **Keppra**, or **Versed** (a nasal spray).
- If you don't have above meds in the home but have **Ativan**, dissolve in a tiny amount of water and squirt into side of mouth.
- Call nurse or MD for support.

SUDDEN SEVERE PAIN

Sudden, severe pain is rare. It usually requires healthcare professionals, but there are things you can do immediately. If the patient is not on hospice, you probably will need to call 911 for support.

Causes:

- Heart attack, or lack of circulation to the heart, can cause chest pain (angina) and often the pain travels to the jaw, arms, and back. It is described as "a heavy crushing pain" or "a giant weight on the chest."
- Internal bleeding from organ or blood vessel rupture
- Clots to the lungs can result in pain and severe shortness of breath.
- Clots to the brain vary from extreme headache to stroke symptoms, which include loss of speech and weakness on one side of the body.
- Fracture

What can I do for sudden severe pain?

1. Call nurse or doctor.
2. Stay calm and talk to the patient in a soft, reassuring voice. Tell her you're getting help.

Medications for Sudden Severe Pain:

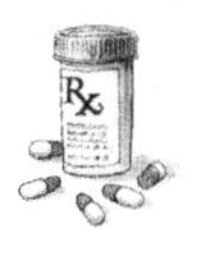

- **Heart attack: Nitroglycerin** is the drug of choice, followed by **morphine or other fast acting opioid.**
- **Severe difficulty breathing: Morphine** or other opioid and **Ativan** for anxiety. Give oxygen if the patient has it.
- **Extreme headache and stroke symptoms: Morphine** for pain and **Ativan** for anxiety.
- **Internal bleeding: Morphine** (This may require more pain control measures, such as a pain pump.)

SWALLOWING DIFFICULTIES/THROAT SECRETIONS

Swallowing is a complex neurological mechanism that is difficult for the body as it gets weaker and weaker.

Causes:

- As patients near death, swallowing becomes hard and choking may occur.
- Mouth sores
- Dry mouth
- Tumor in throat or mouth
- End-stage dementias
- Neurological diseases, like ALS and Parkinson's.

What can I do for swallowing difficulties and excessive secretions?

1. Thickened fluids, such as fruit nectars and milkshakes, are easier to swallow than water.
2. Foods with an applesauce texture are easier to swallow than solid foods.
3. For patients who still want to eat, add gravy and sauces to moisten foods.
4. If the patient can no longer swallow, do not try to feed her anymore, as choking risk is high.
5. For excessive secretions, keep head in raised position, or way over one side in bed to help secretions drain out. May use gentle suction or remove secretions with toothette or turkey baster.

Medications for Swallowing Difficulties

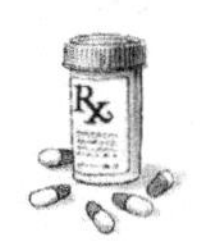

- If mouth sores or painful tumors are the cause, swish with **Miracle Mouthwash** (equal parts **Maalox, Benadryl,** and **Lidocaine**) before eating.
- For thick secretions, use **Mucinex** or **guaifenesin syrup.**
- Medications to dry up secretions: **Robinul, atropine drops** in mouth, **scopolamine patch.**

SWELLING IN FEET, LEGS, AND BELLY

Some diseases can cause fluid to accumulate in different spaces throughout the body and can be very uncomfortable.

Causes of swelling in feet, legs, and belly:

- Heart disease
- Kidney disease
- Liver disease
- Blood clots
- Tumors that block veins and lymphatic channels trapping fluids

What can I do for feet and leg swelling (peripheral edema)?

1. Have patient lie down and elevate legs on pillow.
2. The patient might want to use support hose.
3. If legs are really full and the skin is tight, fluids might leak out of the pores. Call the nurse. You may need to wrap the legs with dressings or absorbent baby diapers.
4. Also watch for redness and pain, which may indicate cellulitis, which is an infection of the skin. The patient may need an antibiotic.

Medications for feet and leg swelling:

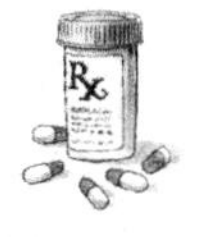

- Use diuretics, such as **Lasix**, as prescribed, to remove excess fluid.

Sudden Swelling in One Leg

If there is sudden swelling and pain in one leg only, it may be a clot. Call your healthcare provider immediately!

ABDOMINAL SWELLING (ASCITES)

This swelling is caused by an accumulation of liquid in the abdominal cavity, most often from liver disease and tumors blocking circulation.

Medications for abdominal swelling:

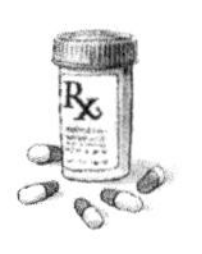

- **Diuretics** can sometimes remove extra fluid.
- Treat symptoms caused by the pressure—such as pain and difficulty breathing—with pain medications, oxygen, and **Ativan.**

What else can be done for abdominal swelling:

- Abdominal tap (paracentesis) The doctor removes fluid by inserting a needle and draining it out. This provides temporary relief, but the abdomen probably will fill back up. (Lung space can also be tapped to remove extra fluid.) Pleurx catheter is sometimes surgically inserted into the chest or abdominal space and left in to drain periodically while the patient is at home.

URINATION: DIFFICULT AND/OR PAINFUL

Urination problems fall into two basic areas:

1. Retention, which is when there is difficulty emptying the bladder
2. Urinary tract infections (UTI) which include the following symptoms: burning sensation, cramping, peeing a small amount at a time, blood in the urine, lower back pain over kidneys, foul smelling and cloudy urine, fever or chills, confusion, incontinence.

Causes:

- Retention problems can be from diseases, like prostate or bladder cancer, or the side effects of medications, like morphine, or end of life weakness.
- Poor hygiene can cause a UTI.
- Catheters and urinary retention put patients at higher risk for infection.
- Painful urination can be caused by a urinary tract infection (UTI), which is a fairly common problem in the dying patient.

Medications for difficult or painful urination:

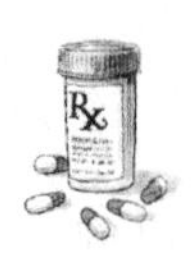

- If infection is suspected (pain, foul smell, fever, confusion, blood in urine, peeing only a little at a time), call your health care provider for a possible antibiotic. In the meantime **pyridium** can be prescribed for pain.
- For retention—first try to get your patient to a toilet/commode and run water in the sink or put a warm washcloth over her bladder area. If she still can't go and is starting to be agitated, feel pain, and her lower abdomen is distended, she most likely needs a catheter
- Call your healthcare provider.

TEN

PAIN—THE BIGGEST FEAR

Not all dying people have pain, yet people fear unrelieved pain more than they fear death itself. As a caregiver, the ultimate priority should be good pain control. This means giving the best medication at the right time.

LIVING AS PAIN FREE AS POSSIBLE

This chapter is a complete guide to pain: what causes it and what you, the caregiver can do to make your patient's life as pain-free as possible. We don't assume that you have a medicine cabinet full of prescription drugs, but we do believe it's important for caregivers to understand the meds that can help their patient and be able to discuss options with the healthcare provider.

Katie
The number one goal in my line of business is good pain control. The first question I ask when I walk through the door of a patient's home is, 'Are you comfortable?' If the patient is in pain everything else goes out the window. He can't eat. He can't get his affairs in order. He can't enjoy visitors or even communicate with loved ones.

The Four Basic Principles of Good Pain Control

1. If a patient says she's hurting, she's hurting.
2. Each person's pain must be treated individually.
3. Everyone has the right to have his pain relieved and to stay as mentally clear as possible.
4. A person should be involved in her pain meds plan, as much as possible.

ASSESSING PAIN

Jahnna

When I asked Dad, "Are you in pain," he'd say, in his Okie accent, "I'm suffering from every pain known to medical science." But it was difficult to find out what hurt and what kind of pain he had. So I'd ask questions like:

1. Can you point to where it hurts?
2. On a scale of zero to 10, what number is your pain?
3. Is your pain mild, moderate or severe?
4. Does your pain come and go or do you have it all the time?
5. Is it all over? Is it an achy pain? Does it burn? Do you feel shooting pain?
6. What has been helpful to alleviate the pain so far?
7. What makes your pain worse?

Dad would finally point to his hip and say, "I ache here. And my legs ache."

SIGNS OF PHYSICAL PAIN

When asked if they hurt, some people may say no for various reasons. They don't want to be a bother or seem weak. Or they have been conditioned to be stoical about pain. Some think if they ignore the pain, it will go away. Whatever the reason, look for physical signs that reveal the patient's discomfort. Try using alternative words and phrases like, "Are you uncomfortable? What can I do to make you more comfortable? Do you have any aches?" Here are seven signs of pain:

1. **Verbal expressions** or sounds such as "I hurt!" "Ow!" "Help!" Whimpering sounds.
2. **Facial expressions:** Grimaces, frowns, eyes squeezed shut, pursed lips, gritted teeth.
3. **Body language:** Stiffening of body, curling up in a ball, pulling away when touched, or reaching out. Holding breath or holding the body in a frozen position.
4. **Physiological:** Increase in blood pressure and pulse, sweaty, clammy skin; lack of appetite. Heavy or increased breathing.
5. **Social:** Loss of interest in activities or people. Withdrawn.
6. **Emotional:** Irritable, angry, anxious, depressed.
7. **Spiritual:** Questioning and blaming God, feeling victimized, guilty, and hopeless.

FALSE BELIEFS ABOUT PAIN

- Pain is a punishment for my sins.
- If I admit I'm in pain, I'll be seen as weak.
- I should take medication only when the pain gets bad.
- If I take strong medications now, they won't work later.
- People who are sleeping or in a coma don't experience pain.
- It will go away if I just ignore it.

Chronic Pain

People with chronic pain may not show a lot of the physical signs because they are used to it.

PAIN CONTROL

How to avoid pain: take medicine on schedule!

A patient should not wait until the pain returns to take the medication. Otherwise, he'll feel pain, take the meds, and then have to wait for 30 to 45 minutes for the medicine to move into his bloodstream. Staying on schedule will make the patient feel better about everything—activities, eating, and living.

Addressing Pain: Not all Pain is the same

Most of the pain that people experience in their lives is somatic, or general pain, caused by things like cutting their finger, breaking an arm, or arthritis.

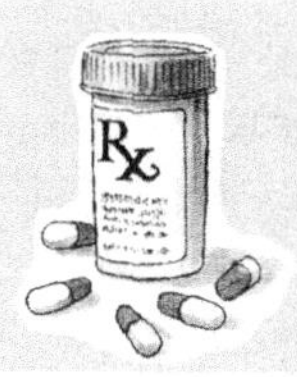

When you see this image, a doctor or nurse must first be consulted before administering any of the prescription medicines mentioned in this chapter.

SOMATIC PAIN (General Pain) can be easily identified. For example: when you stub your toe, you know exactly where it hurts, and what it feels like. Somatic pain is often described as a sharp, stabbing, throbbing, or aching pain.

What causes somatic pain?

- Injuries to the skin, muscles, tendons, ligaments, and bones
- Arthritis
- Accidents, wounds, skin infections and sores
- Migraines and cluster headaches
- Muscle tears and sprains
- Bone fractures
- Inactivity

Medications for somatic pain:

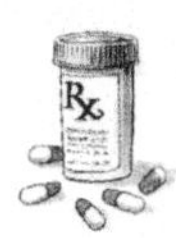

- This kind of specific pain is usually very easy to treat. It responds very well to pain medications that range from **Tylenol** and **Advil** to **morphine.**

BONE PAIN is a specific type of somatic pain that most commonly presents itself as a constant dull, deep ache that worsens with activity.

What causes bone pain?

- Bone cancer
- Fractures
- Multiple myeloma, which is a bone marrow cancer
- Bone metastasis, or bone "mets," where the cancer starts somewhere else, and spreads to the spine, pelvis, or the long bones of the legs or arms.

Medications commonly used for bone pain:

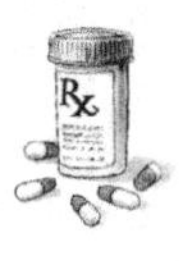

- Over the counter anti-inflammatory drugs such as **Advil** or **Aleve**
- Steroid drugs, like **prednisone** and **Decadron**, are very powerful anti-inflammatories.
- Opioids such as **Norco** can be used as pain increases.
- Short-term doses of radiation to tumors may relieve bone pain.

Jahnna
When Dad's prostate cancer moved to his bones he had agonizing back pain. One doctor prescribed a series of narcotics that only made him goofy. He was afraid his lift chair was out to get him and he kept trying to exit the house through the fireplace. But his pain was still there. Katie suggested we try an anti-inflammatory to help with the tumors pressing on the spine. We gave him three Advil twice a day and it was like a miracle—the pain in his back almost disappeared. And we were able to significantly lower his narcotic dose. (He was happily back in his lift chair and when he left the house he went through the front door!)

NERVE PAIN is the most difficult pain to treat. It feels like a constant burning, often with sudden episodes of shooting pain or electrical shock sensations.

What causes nerve pain?

- Cancer, diabetes, and chemotherapy can cause peripheral neuropathy—a burning pain in the hands and feet.
- Tumors
- Scar tissue from surgery
- Radiation
- Direct damage to nerve tissues or from nerves being compressed
- Shingles, which is a reactivation of the chicken pox virus that occurs when a person's immune system is compromised. It travels along the nerve pathways.

Nerve pain may worsen with exposure to heat or cold, or contact with clothing or bed sheets, or simply touching the areas near the location of the pain.

Medications commonly used for nerve pain

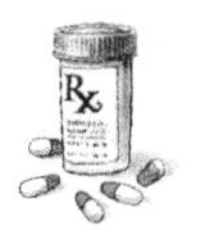

- Seizure drugs, like **Neurontin** and **Tegretol** suppress the abnormal nerve signals that cause nerve pain. (Some people can't tolerate these medications because they get dizzy or feel too sedated.)
- Antidepressants such as **Elavil** can stimulate the body's natural pain relieving mechanisms and help increase the effects of narcotics like **morphine.** This medication does not relieve pain right away and must be taken steadily for two to three days before it kicks in. It also has the good side effects of helping depression and sleeping problems, so you want to give it at night. Sometimes **Pamelor** is used because Elavil makes some people too sleepy.
- For shingles, antiviral medicines, such as **Acyclovir** and **Famciclovir,** can reduce the pain and duration of the outbreak. **Caladryl** lotion also helps relieve pain.

VISCERAL PAIN (Organ Pain) is often described as cramping or spasms in the liver, intestines, stomach, and other organs. The pain often radiates to other parts of the abdomen or back. It can feel like a tight band around a person's mid-section or up-under-the-rib pain.

What causes visceral pain?

- A tumor that invades an organ or blocks a passage-way between organs
- Swollen or distended organs
- A blocked bowel, which can result in severe nausea and vomiting

Medications commonly used for visceral pain:

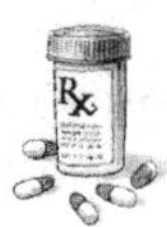

- **Atropine,** (which is used in eye drops), and **scopolamine** (often used for sea sickness) have been found to be very effective in relieving cramping pain.
- **Levsin,** a smooth muscle relaxer, also helps with spasms and cramping.
- **Belladonna** and **opium** suppositories are sometimes used for rectal and pelvic pain.
- **Steroids** help reduce the swelling around a tumor, which can relieve visceral pain.

SUDDEN, SEVERE PAIN

Sudden, severe pain is rare. It usually requires health care professionals, but there are things you can do immediately. If the patient is not on hospice, you probably will need to call 911 for support.

What causes sudden, severe pain:

- Heart attack
- Clots to the lungs or brain
- Bone fracture
- Internal bleeding from organ or blood vessel rupture.
- Bowel/bladder obstruction

Medications commonly used for sudden, severe pain

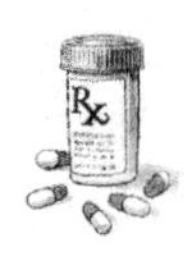

- **Nitroglycerine** opens the blood vessels in a heart attack and **morphine** helps with pain.

Medications commonly used for sudden, severe pain (continued)

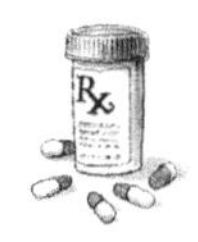

- **Morphine** and **Ativan** for difficulty breathing, extreme headaches and stroke symptoms associated with clots to the lungs and brain.
- Pain pump if the pain is severe.

MORPHINE—THE GOLD STANDARD OF PAIN CONTROL

Morphine mimics our own endorphins naturally released by the brain whenever we have pain or become excited. Endorphins relieve pain by binding directly to the brain's pain receptors. As pain worsens, our natural endorphins are no longer adequate, and we must turn to **morphine** and other opioids, like **Dilaudid** or **Oxycodone**, for help.

Morphine is delivered in several forms:

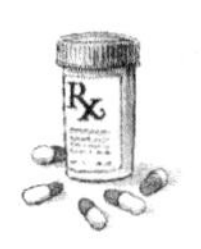

- **Fast-acting tabs or liquids (morphine sulfate)** can be used separately or in combination with long-acting morphine for "breakthrough" pain, which is pain that may flare up between long-acting doses. The liquid can be swallowed, or given slowly under the tongue, or in the cheek if a patient is unable to swallow. A single dose should last about 4 hours, but can be given more frequently for breakthrough pain.
- **Time-release pills: MS Contin (oramorph)** is a long-acting pain release tablet given every 8–to–12 hours on a regular schedule. Small and easy to swallow, it can also be given rectally.
- **Patient-controlled pump: Liquid morphine sulfate** is delivered by an IV tube in a vein, or a soft catheter under the skin. It provides a steady infusion of medication and patients push a button for extra doses when they need it. These battery-operated pumps are small and allow people to remain mobile, and the pump is preprogrammed so that there is no risk of overdose.

Synthetic Opioids:

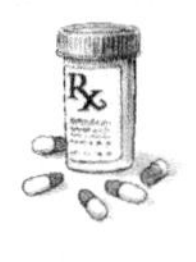

- **Oxycodone** is a fast-acting pill or liquid. Generally it has fewer gastrointestinal side effects than morphine.

Synthetic Opioids (continued):

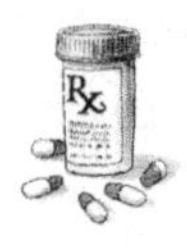

- **Oxycontin** is the time-release form of Oxycodone.
- **Duragesic (fentanyl)** is a pain patch applied to the upper arms, back, or chest. It provides a constant dose of pain medication through the skin, and is changed every 72 hours. It takes 12–to–16 hours for the first one to reach full effect. Fever or heat (electric blankets, hot weather, etc.) speeds up the absorption rate, so the patch may need to be changed sooner.

- **Dilaudid (hydromorphone)** comes in liquid, pill, suppository or IV. It also has a time-release form.
- **Methadone** is a long-acting medication in liquid or pill form.

OPIOID SIDE EFFECTS:

Sedation, nausea, itching and constipation generally resolve themselves (except constipation) within a week.

What to do:

- Avoid constipation with stool softeners, stimulants, and juice.
- Use **Zofran** or **Compazine** to deal with nausea.
- If the nausea occurs primarily after eating, along with bloating and loss of appetite, **Reglan** may be more effective.
- Antihistamines, like **Benadryl,** can help relieve itching.

Less common side effects:

- Swollen feet and hands can be treated with diuretics (**Lasix**).
- Jerky movements and twitching can occur, particularly at bedtime or during the evening hours. If severe, treat with mild tranquilizers—**Ativan, Valium,** and **Klonipin**—or change to a different opioid. Or rotate them.
- Occasionally, people become confused and hallucinate. These side effects often resolve on their own. If not, talk to your health care provider who may suggest adding other meds or backing off the opioids.

Opioids and Urinary Retention

Morphine and other opioids may make it difficult to empty the bladder (urinary retention.) This is more common in males, especially those with prostate problems. If this becomes severe, a catheter may be needed.

FEARS ABOUT MORPHINE

In Katie's 24 years as a hospice social worker, these are the most common questions asked about morphine.

My wife doesn't want to be all doped up. Won't morphine make her confused?
If she's on the right dose, this shouldn't be a problem. Some patients become more alert because they're more comfortable. Occasionally, the drug may cause sedation and mild confusion, but this usually resolves within a week. In rare cases, someone may experience mild hallucinations. These usually go away, too.

If my dad starts taking Morphine now, will it work later?
Your health care provider or nurse will help you adjust the dose, as you need it. There's no upper limit to the amount of morphine you can use.

Does morphine make you constipated?
Yes. Pain medicine can cause your bowels to slow down. Constipation will occur if you don't have a bowel plan, which includes stool softeners and laxatives. This is no reason to refuse morphine, because this side effect is easily controlled.

I'm afraid to give my mother morphine. What if I overdose her?
The morphine binds to the pain receptors in the brain. As long as your mother is having symptoms, like pain or shortness of breath, you will not overdose her. You can give your loved one as much as needed to make her comfortable, per doctor's direction.

Will morphine kill my husband?
No. Morphine is simply one of the best medications for pain. Sometimes patients require a lot of morphine before they die, but the morphine doesn't kill them. It simply helps them die in comfort. That's the goal.

If the doctor puts my mother on morphine, does it mean she's dying now?
No. Some people are on morphine for months before they die.

Won't morphine make him a drug addict?
If you are using morphine because you are in pain, you will not get addicted. Addicts take it to get high, not because they are in pain. The wife of one of my patients worried that her husband was going to become addicted. He looked at her and said, "Honey, I'm dying. Who cares?" And he was right. The number one objective is pain relief.

HELPER DRUGS

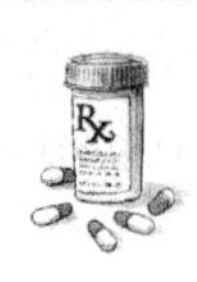

- **Adjuvant or adjunctive drugs** are drugs that are not usually used for pain but may be helpful for its management. They are often used with **morphine** and other **opioids**, to increase or aid their effect.

- **Non steroidal anti-inflammatories or NSAIDS (Advil and Aleve)** help with bone pain and other inflammatory pain, like headaches.
- **Steroids (Prednisone and Decadron)** are powerful anti-inflammatories used for advanced bone pain, severe headaches from increased intra-cranial pressure, brain metastasis, spinal cord compression and cramping in the internal organs.

  Take in the morning with food and add anti-ulcer medications such as **Zantac, Prilosec,** or **Prevacid**. They also can cause elevated blood sugars, so should be used with extreme caution by people with diabetes.

  Side Effects of Steroids:
  Positive side effects from steroids are increased energy and appetite.
  Negative side effects include fluid retention, irritability, agitation, and insomnia. Steroids may cause stomach upset.

- **Anti-seizure medications (Tegretol, Neurontin)** are used for nerve pain.
- **Anti-depressants (Elavil)** are used for nerve pain.

- **Muscle relaxants (Valium, Soma)** are used for spasms or cramps of the skeletal muscles, which are in the legs, arms, back and abdomen **Baclofen** is often used to control spasms caused by multiple sclerosis or spinal cord injuries, and to stop bowel or bladder spasms.
- **Smooth muscle relaxers (Levsin, belladonna and opium suppositories)** help with pain and cramping in the organs.
- **Diuretics (Lasix)** dry up the extra fluid in the lungs, legs, abdomen, and tissues.
- **Antihistamines (Benadryl and Vistaril)** help relieve itching.
- **Atropine and Levsin** are used for spasms and cramping of the smooth muscles, which are in the intestines, liver, pancreas, gall bladder, and all the internal organs.
- **Nitroglycerin** is used for angina, or heart pain.

PLO (Pluronic Lecithin Organogel)

Many medications can be put into gels or creams. It is applied to the skin and absorbed into the bloodstream. Meds that can be administered this way are: **ibuprofen, Ativan, Haldol, Neurontin,** and some **opioids.**

- PLOs are especially useful for people who have sensitive stomachs or cannot swallow.
- These gels are also good for patients with dementia and Alzheimer's who are combative and refuse to take medication.
- PLOs can offer localized pain control for arthritis.

MORE ADVANCED OPTIONS FOR PAIN CONTROL

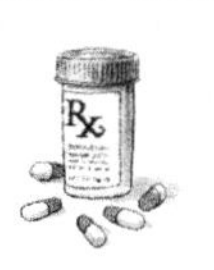

- **A Nerve Block is an injection of narcotics, steroids, or anti-inflammatories,** into various parts of the body. One example is an epidural block, which can be a single injection or a continuous infusion, via a pump, into the epidural space of the spine.

Advanced Options for Pain Control (Continued)

Radiation can shrink cancer tumors, taking the pressure off organs and nerves.

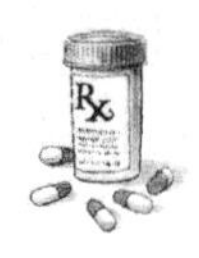

- **Palliative Sedation** keeps the patient in a sleep-like state for her remaining days or hours. It is used when a patient's pain or symptoms cannot be controlled, even on high doses of opioids. (Patients usually have advanced metastatic cancer.) A pump administers drugs, such as **Versed,** intravenously or subcutaneously. The patient dies from the terminal disease or condition NOT from the infusion. Sometimes rectal meds, such as **phenobarbital** or **Thorazine**, are used.

ALTERNATIVE PAIN RELIEF

Medical marijuana (cannabis), at this writing, is legal for medical use in 18 states, and 7 of these states allow dispensaries to sell it. Some of the established benefits are in the treatment of:

- nausea and vomiting
- loss of appetite
- insomnia
- muscle spasms
- nerve pain
- Multiple Sclerosis
- ALS

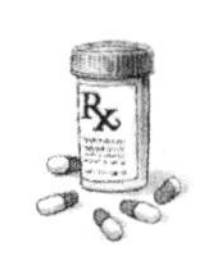

- In the US, oral pills are **Marinol, Canasol,** and **Nabilone.** Besides pill form, cannabis can be administered by vaporizing or smoking the dried buds, oils, drinking or eating extracts (in muffins, butter, brownies, etc.), and taking capsules.

NON-MEDICAL PAIN RELIEF

There are options to use in conjunction with medications or alone.

- **Hot or Cold Therapy**
  A hot water bottle or heating pad can provide relief to sore, stiff muscles or crampy-feeling places. If the patient is able, a soak in a hot tub or bath can be relaxing and improve circulation. Cold packs are not used as often as heat, but they are beneficial if the cause of pain is from a fall or injury.

- **Massage** is wonderful for stiff and achy bodies. We all get sore when we are in the same position too long, even if we're just sitting in a chair. Most people can tolerate a gentle back or foot rub.

- **Aromatherapy**
  Use essential oils to enhance psychological and physical well-being. Lemon oil has been found to reduce stress. Lavender, Jasmine, and Peppermint are used for anxiety, stress, and depression. Put a few drops on the pillow, or in a diffuser, or use in massage oils.

- **Meditation and Guided Imagery**
  Pain is both physically and emotionally stressful, and stress can make the pain worse. Planned, purposeful relaxation can reduce stress and therefore reduce pain and add to a feeling of well-being. For some simple exercises for meditation and guided imagery, see Chapter 3, pg. 27.

Specialists

- **Acupuncture** dates back more than 3,000 years. It involves insertion of needles into specific points in the body where energy is believed to be blocked. When the energy that runs through these channels is out of balance, people may be more prone to pain. Acupuncture is meant to restore the balance and help a variety of conditions, including pain, stress, and fluid build-up.

- **Reflexology** is the practice of applying pressure to the feet and hands using specific thumb, finger, and hand techniques, without the use of lotions. The belief is that certain areas in the hands and the feet correspond to an organ, or area, of the body. Applying pressure to these specific areas can provide pain relief.

Remember

"Pain is whatever the person says it is, existing whenever they say it does."

—Margo McCaffery,
pioneer in the field of pain

Part Three

JOURNEY'S END

ELEVEN

HOW WE DIE

What to Expect in the Last Months, Weeks, Days, and Hours of Life

PREPARING TO GO

The process of dying can be compared to the labor of being born. Some people go through the labor of death in months. Some in days, or even hours. Some people start the process years before, when dying is from old age. Though every death is different, there are similarities that occur in the dying process. Knowing what to expect in the last weeks, days, and hours can lessen some of the fear for the patient and the caregiver.

The Body's Plan

Our body really does know how to die itself. It has a system for shutting down that is kind and helps us have a good death. It's pretty straightforward—the closer we get to death, the less we want to eat or drink. This is not painful because the body releases endorphins and ketones, which are natural painkillers that cause mild euphoria and sedation.

Dehydration is not painful.

It is normal in the dying process and may actually add to the comfort of the patient. As the body dehydrates there is less fluid in the lungs and heart to cause congestion. There is less pressure around tumors, so pain may decrease. Dehydration leads to electrolyte imbalance causing a release of chemicals that make us sleepy. And peaceful.

Each Death is Unique

People tend to die the way they lived. They handle the challenge of dying the way they handled other challenges in their lives:

- People who ran away from their problems in life tend to deny that they are dying, sometimes even up to the very end.
- People who were controlling types will orchestrate their dying down to who they want in the room, and what music they want playing, and make sure it happens that way.
- The protective mother will not die with her children in the room. She'll let them sit by the bedside for 24 hours, and in the five minutes they take to go to the bathroom, she'll choose to die.
- If a person has been a fighter his entire life, challenging everyone and everything, he will probably go out fighting.

THE LABOR OF DEATH

There are three stages to the labor of death: **Early, transitional,** and **active labor.** In each stage there are things you can do to help your loved one stay comfortable.

EARLY LABOR: ONE TO FOUR MONTHS BEFORE DEATH

- Lack of energy and major fatigue
- Decrease in appetite
- Withdrawal from the world

Lack of Energy and Major Fatigue

- Your loved one tires faster.
- He may start taking an afternoon nap, and then add a morning and evening nap.
- Outings and activities decrease or stop.
- Increased time is spent in bed or dozing in a chair.

What can I do?

1. Pace patient's activities to conserve energy.
2. Limit the number of visitors and length of visits.
3. Naps are totally okay. You don't need to wake the patient.
4. Use this time to share more quiet activities: watch movies, look at photos, and listen to music.

Decrease in Appetite and Eating

- Patient starts to refuse certain foods. Usually meat first, then vegetables. He says things like, "Nothing tastes good."
- Patient tires after a few bites.
- The body is starting to reject food.

The patient may want to eat to please others, but "Just can't." It's normal to lose the desire to eat because the body can't digest food the way it used to. Offering big meals can be overwhelming and cause constipation, nausea, and bloating. Be careful of equating food with love.

Jahnna
In the beginning, Mom's daily report was all about the food she got Dad to eat. She'd be thrilled when he ate a six-course meal: meatballs, broccoli, salad, rice, some ice cream, and cookies. As the months passed, Mom finally figured out that Dad didn't need or want all that food, and offered a small bowl of soup or cup of yogurt, and that was enough.

What can I do?

1. Remember, at this time, food is more for comfort than nutrition.
2. Offer small amounts of food. Offer, but don't force!
3. Cool, creamy foods like yogurt, pudding, smoothies or milk-shakes go down easier.
4. Patients enjoy mashed potatoes and gravy, or soft-boiled eggs.
5. Baby food can be spiced up to be tasty.
6. You might want to share a chocolate mousse or a bowl of ice cream as more of a social event, than an eating event.
7. Speaking of ice cream—if a patient only wants to eat ice cream let him!

What if the Patient has Feeding Tube?

His desire and need for food will decrease over time, just as if he were eating. The rule is: go by what the patient is feeling and what his body is telling him. When the patient starts developing symptoms such as nausea, bloating, diarrhea, and choking–those are signs to decrease the amount. As he gets close to dying, you can continue to give feeding in small amounts, if he says he's hungry. Usually a few days before the patient dies, the feeding is stopped completely because at this time it's doing more harm then good. Fluid may even collect in the lungs, making extra work for the body.

Patient May Start to Withdraw from the World

Detaching and withdrawal is normal. Your loved one is starting to loosen the ties that bind her to this world. The focus is now turned inwards where she's quietly examining her life and doing the hard work of dying.

- Patient begins losing interest in outside activities, social life, newspapers, and TV.
- She may become quieter and talk less.
- She may start refusing company.
- Though awake, she may have her eyes closed.
- She may prefer to be alone.

What can I do?

1. Don't take this detachment personally. She is preparing to take the biggest trip of her life and there is a lot to figure out.
2. Allow your loved one the quiet time alone, but don't abandon her.
3. Limit visitors. Ask first before anyone comes.
4. Keep reassuring the patient that you are there if she needs you.

Jahnna

Dad stopped wanting visitors and didn't enjoy talking on the phone. What he did enjoy was the time he spent with his caregiver who played the guitar. They sang songs together almost to the last day.

TRANSITIONAL LABOR: ONE TO TWO WEEKS BEFORE DEATH

- Sleeping increases and eating decreases
- May be confused and disoriented
- May talk in travel metaphors about having to go somewhere.
- May start seeing people in the room.

Sleeping Increases and Eating Decreases

- He may stop eating all together, only taking fluids.
- The patient is probably in the bed or a recliner all of the time.
- He is sleeping more than he is awake, sometimes with his mouth open and his eyes not quite closed.

What can I do?

1. Think about the atmosphere the patient would want. He may want to have his favorite music playing or the TV off. Or on. Some people like hearing the familiar family noises where others prefer quiet.
2. Reposition the patient every few hours in the daytime.
3. Use pillows to support knees, back, and in between the legs.
4. Check bony areas for red spots; reposition patient as needed.
5. Continue to offer liquids. If he has difficulty swallowing, offer thicker substances like a spoonful of pudding or applesauce, which are easier to swallow than water or juice.

Patient May be Confused and Disoriented

- He looses track of days and time.
- He may be confused about where he is and who is with him.
- He confuses dreams with reality.
- He may "pick" at bed sheets and clothes or the space in front of him.

What can I do?

In the last week of life, most patients get disoriented because their world has become so small—they loose track of time and place. The anchors they had in the world are disappearing. Be calm, play soothing music, and reassure them they're fine. (If they become really agitated, it could be caused by a full bladder.)

Patients May Start Seeing People in the Room

- He may see things and people who are not there.
- Some patients see angels or Jesus.
- He may talk with people or relatives who have already died.

Jahnna

Two weeks before he died, Dad started seeing a man who stood to the left of his chair. He'd carry on whispered conversations with him, laughing and nodding. He'd even cup his hand around his mouth, so we wouldn't hear them talking. Three days before he died, Dad asked me to peek behind him and see if that man was still there. I said, "Yes," and he smiled and said, "Good."

What can I do?

1. Don't argue with the patient or deny what he is seeing.
2. He is really living more in the world of his dreams than this world and that's perfectly normal.

Katie
Arlene kept seeing a man on a dark horse coming for her. She asked her daughter to, "Tell that man to go away." Arlene's daughter firmly told the horseman, "Go away. My mother does not want you here." Arlene, who had been so agitated, immediately calmed down and the horseman disappeared.

Medications for agitation

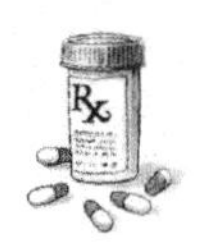

- If his visions are disturbing and persist, or he gets agitated or afraid, there are medications, like **Ativan** or **Haldol**, that can help.

Jahnna
A few days before he died, Dad suddenly had to get out of bed. He was frantic. He needed to get to his funeral. People were waiting and he was late. Dad's caregiver finally helped him out of bed and wheeled him into the living room where Dad greeted a room full of people that only he could see. He tried to get to his feet to address them, but lost strength and sat back in the chair, exhausted from his effort.

Patient May Talk in Metaphors About Having to Go Somewhere

- A lot of patients say, "I want to go home." And their families respond, "But you are home." They're actually talking about going to their ultimate home.
- Many patients use travel metaphors like, "I have to catch a bus," or "a plane."
- Others suddenly have to pack or get dressed.

Katie
The day before my father died, he kept talking about needing to get on a ship. He kept asking, "Who's going to be the captain and drive the boat?" My sisters and I reassured him that we would get him to the boat. And I volunteered to drive it to where he needed to go. He died with his eyes wide open, gazing out at the ocean.

What can I do?
Once again don't argue, just go along with him, like Katie did when her father was dying.

What Keeps Us Here?

Some patients struggle with leaving. They have a long drawn-out end to their life. There are three basic reasons why people may have a hard time parting from this world:

1. Pain creates a tension that traps us in our body. We need to relax to die. It's why hospice medicates people until they die, even if they're unresponsive.
2. Anger and Fear are powerful emotions. Fear of "not going to heaven," or anger about having to die.
3. Unfinished business in relationships. When people die, they never worry that they didn't spend enough time at the their jobs. They worry about the amount of time spent with loved ones and words that need to be said.

ACTIVE LABOR: A FEW DAYS TO HOURS BEFORE DEATH

- Patient is mostly unresponsive in a semi-comatose state
- Blood pressure decreases and pulse increases
- Breathing changes
- Temperature changes
- Circulation and skin changes
- Some may have a sudden surge of energy and call out.
- Can no longer swallow

Patient is Mostly Unresponsive in a Semi-Comatose State

- The patient's eyes become glazed, not focusing
- Often the patient sleeps with her eyes and mouth slightly open

What can I do?

1. Sit by the bed. The patient knows you are there.
2. Continue to talk to the patient. Though she may be unresponsive, she can still hear you. Tell her that she's doing a good job.
3. Reassure the patient that you will be okay, and if she needs to go, she can.
4. This is a chance to say whatever it is that needs to be said.
5. Hearing is the last sense to go. Soft music or prayers are comforting.

Katie

Sue was actively dying but fighting it with everything she had. Though mostly asleep, when she was awake she was either moaning or crying (not because of physical pain) and fighting with the caregivers, spitting her medication at them. She had a terrible relationship with her children. Because of a lifetime of wrongs done to them, they really did not want to see or even speak to her. But the night before Sue died, her daughter showed up at her bedside. She kissed her mother on the cheek and said, "Mom, I'm here. It's all about love now." Sue's breathing suddenly quieted and a tear rolled down her cheek. She died peacefully during the night.

Breathing Changes

- Breathing may vary at this time—sometimes rapid, up to 50 breaths a minute, and sometimes deep and labored.
- Patient may have stop-and-start breathing (apneic breathing)
- Breathing can stop for up to a minute and then start up again.
- Jaw may drop open as the patient mouth breathes.
- Saliva and mucous may increase in the back of the throat because the patient is unable to cough and swallow.
- Mucous may increase, creating a loud "death rattle" in the throat.
- Secretions may even become copious and frothy, especially in patients with heart failure.

What can I do?

1. Raise the head of the bed. For most, it's easier to breathe sitting up.
2. Position the patient on her side to decrease secretions.

Clearing the Throat

Suction is not generally advised because it can irritate the back of the throat and encourages more saliva and mucous. But if there is a big build-up in the patient's cheek, a turkey-baster, or ear bulb, may be able to get rid of some of it.

Blood Pressure Decreases and Pulse Increases

- This is normal and expected.

Medications for the final hours:

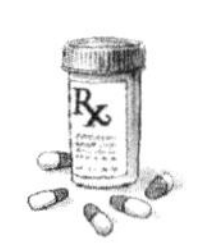

- Medications, like **atropine** or a **scopolamine** patch can help dry up the secretions.
- If secretions are copious and frothy a dose of **Lasix** may help.
- For pain and labored breathing, medications like **morphine** and **Ativan** can bring relief.
- If the patient is very close to death, you may want to remove the oxygen to make it easier for her to go. Most of the time it is no longer needed.

Temperature Changes

- Temperature can swing from hot to cold.
- Patient may break out in a sweaty fever.
- Skin may get clammy and develop a yellowish color.

What can I do?

1. Dress the patient in a loose cotton gown or tee shirt, and if he's hot, remove the covers. If he's cold, adjust accordingly.
2. Patient may prefer to be naked, so remove clothes.

Do Not Use Electric Blanket or Heating Pad

The patient's temperature is too unpredictable and you might end up overheating him or burning his skin, which can be ultra-sensitive because of poor circulation.

If Feverish:

1. Place a cool washcloth on his forehead.
2. Offer small sips of water every couple of hours, if patient can swallow. Otherwise use toothettes.
3. Give a light sponge bath with lukewarm water.
4. You can use Tylenol to reduce temperature (rectally if the patient cannot swallow).

Circulation and Skin Changes

- Hands and feet may become very cold because the heart can't circulate normally.
- When you hold the patient's hand, she may no longer respond.
- A red mottling may develop around the knees, on the chest, and across the back.
- As the patient drinks less water, the body gets dehydrated and pulls fluid from the lungs, around the heart, the feet, hands, and belly.
- A dark blue coloring may appear on her feet, knees, hands, and around the mouth.

What can I do?

1. Understand this discoloration is normal.
2. Keep a light blanket or sheet over the patient's body and apply lip balm as needed.

Patient May Have a Sudden Surge of Energy and Call Out

- Some patients, after days of sleeping, may have a surge of energy, wanting to get up and talk and even eat.
- Some, who have been sleeping for days, may suddenly sit up and make an announcement.
- Patients may see people they know waiting for them, and even call them by name.
- A patient may have a period of agitation or restlessness, trying to get up, yelling out, "I have to go!" or "Mama!"
- As mentioned earlier, the patient may speak in travel metaphors. But now it is more urgent. "I have to catch a train." Or "The plane is about to leave. I have to go!"

Patient Can No Longer Swallow

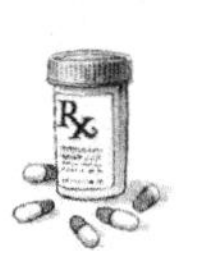

1. Talk to the nurse about giving only medicines that don't have to be swallowed.
2. Increase medications, like **Ativan** or **morphine**, as needed for breathing difficulty or pain.
3. Provide mouth care regularly—about every 2 to 3 hours: use toothettes or swabs to moisten mouth and lip balm for dry lips.

4. Add a few drops of vegetable oil to the water glass before dipping in the toothette. It helps keep the mouth moist.
5. You may also drop small amounts of water or ice chips in the mouth with a syringe or straw, but just enough to coat the mouth so the person doesn't choke.
6. Some people clench their jaws tight, making it difficult to get inside their mouths, so just use a toothette around their teeth, doing the best you can. Don't force the jaw open.

Some People Choose to Die Alone

Some people choose to die alone, just as some wait for family to arrive. You may have been sitting by the bed for three hours, and when you step out of the room just a minute or two, that's when your loved one slips away. Don't be hard on yourself if this happens. It was a choice your loved one made. It may have been easier for her to leave when she was alone.

JUST BEFORE DEATH

- Patients may start "guppy breathing," which sounds like faint, gasping breaths and looks like a fish out of water.
- Quite often the patient's body stiffens and her face may grimace slightly. Then she will take a breath or two more, and be gone.
- Often the patient is very peaceful and calm and the moment of death is barely noticeable, except for the cessation of breathing.

People Fear Bladder or Bowel Will Release Upon Death

This doesn't necessarily happen. By the time of death, a patient has usually stopped drinking and eating, and his bowel and bladder are pretty empty.

THE MOMENT OF DEATH

- Some people grimace or frown before their final two or three breaths. Some may even smile.
- It's not a grimace of pain, it's more of a preparation for the letting go of life.

DEATH: HOW DO WE KNOW HE IS DEAD?

- Breathing has stopped for several minutes and the heart has stopped.
- If his eyelids are open, the eyes will remain in a fixed stare.
- The jaw may drop open.
- Color gradually leaves the person's face.
- The body cools down and stiffens over several hours.

Jahnna
Katie and I had just checked on Dad. His hands and feet were blue, there was a red-looking rash on his knee joints and chest, traveling from his heart to his throat. His eyes were closed and he was breathing fast but not panting. We went back to the living room and suddenly there was a lot of static over the baby monitor. Katie turned to me and said, "He's gone." At 6:20 the sun set and took Dad with it.

What do I do at the moment of death?

- You don't have to do anything right away, simply be in the sacred moment.
- Gently close your loved one's eyes and prop his head up on a pillow to close his jaw.
- If you are planning on having a viewing, slip the patient's dentures into his mouth.
- When you feel ready, call hospice, if the patient is on hospice. If the patient was on a medication pump, the nurse or your health care provider will need to come out and remove it.

Katie
After my father, who was an artist, died, my sisters and I dressed him in his signature khaki shirt and khaki pants. My sister shaved him and trimmed his hair for his journey back to his hometown, where he was to be buried. We splashed on his cologne and made sure he had a handkerchief in his pocket.

Who do I call?

- If the patient is not on hospice, call the funeral home. Every state's law is different. The funeral home will know who should be notified.
- If no funeral home has been chosen yet, call the county coroner or police. Tell them it is not an emergency.
- The funeral home will send someone to pick up your loved one. It doesn't have to be right away. You can ask them to wait till morning or in a few hours—after you've had a chance to sit with the body.
- You may choose to bathe and dress your loved one. Put a few drops of lavender oil or other scent in the water.
- If you haven't already picked clothes ahead of time, choose clothing that's easy to put on and has meaning to you or to him, even if it's just a favorite tee shirt.
- Most people would like the body to be removed within a few hours, but there are some people who would like to keep the body at home for a wake and viewing.
- Laws vary from state to state. In Oregon, after 24 hours, you must cool the body if you want to keep it at home. You'll need to place dry ice around the body.

Take Time to Acknowledge the Moment

Once you've made the call to the authorities, put on tea or open a bottle of wine. Light candles. Play music. Have a toast to your loved one and to yourself. Your presence in this journey has been the greatest gift of love.

Jahnna

When Dad died, his face was amazing. The wrinkles were instantly gone. We rolled up a small towel and placed it under his jaw to close it. He looked 30 years younger and was very handsome. Katie had advised us to have clothes ready to put on Dad. Mom chose his B-17 pilot's shirt and sweat pants. (We had pre-cut the shirt up the back to slip on him after he died.) We placed his Glengarry Scottish cap on his head and played his favorite song, "Bring Him Home," from Les Miserables. We all raised a glass of champagne and talked about Dad's amazing exit with the sun. Then we hugged and kissed my father good-bye.

TWELVE

WHAT TO DO AFTER DEATH

Funeral Options and Who to Contact

As a caregiver, you are still running a marathon, but if you have had a chance to prepare for this moment, you will be a little ahead of the game. If you haven't had a chance to make arrangements, now is the time to contact a funeral home and decide if you want a burial or cremation. Now is also the time to ask your friends and family for help.

What you need to do within the week

- ❑ Decide if you want a viewing, a funeral, a graveside service and/or a memorial service.
- ❑ Bring to the funeral home: clothing, cosmetics, glasses, shoes, and anything you would like put in the casket.
- ❑ Choose a funeral/memorial date, taking into consideration the availability of the person you want to officiate and the time it might take for close friends and relatives to travel to the event.
- ❑ If memorial/funeral is not at the funeral home or a church, you may want to make arrangements to rent a hall.
- ❑ Make a list of people who need to know now about your loved one's passing—family, close friends, office, church. Ask a friend or family member to call them for you.
- ❑ Notify organizations: Social Security, the VA, insurance companies, place of employment, retirement/pension funds.
- ❑ Write an obituary.

FUNERAL ARRANGEMENTS

Funeral homes offer a lot of services, but each item costs. And the cost is not cheap. Here is a list of what they can do for you:

- Notify the proper authorities when your loved one dies
- Transfer the deceased to the funeral home
- Put a death notice in the paper with a link to an online obituary
- Help compose an obituary, post it online and put it in the paper with a photo
- Order certified death certificates and copies
- Assist with contacting insurance companies, Social Security, the VA, and help fill out VA paperwork
- Provide acknowledgment cards for family to send out to family and friends

For a Burial (Interment), a funeral home will:

- Bathe, embalm (an option, not necessary), dress, restore, apply cosmetics, and dress hair of the deceased
- Sell you a casket and burial vault (if necessary)
- Provide viewing room and staff to greet visitors, receive flowers at viewing
- Set up guest registry and photo gallery, provide prayer cards
- Make funeral arrangements including arrange for music, contact clergy, and guest speakers
- If the deceased was a veteran, they will contact the VA and arrange for a flag for coffin and a burial in a VA cemetery, if desired
- Order funeral spray and flower arrangements for the memorial service
- Transport body to cemetery
- Transport family to funeral and cemetery and back
- Gather flowers, guest book, memorial contributions, photos, DVDs, and any other items included in the service, and return them to you and your family

For Cremation, a funeral home will:

- Transport the deceased to a crematory
- Provide container for the cremation and an urn for the ashes
- Ship the ashes, if not picked up

What about Direct Cremation?

This is when the body is taken from the place of death directly to the crematory. There is no viewing or service, and no need for a funeral home. The body is cremated in a simple container. This is the most affordable option.

What about a Green Burial?

A green burial allows the body to recycle naturally. The body is buried in a shroud or a biodegradable casket with no metal or concrete lining. The choices go from a simple cardboard casket to a wicker casket. There are some strictly green burial companies, but many funeral homes now offer this option. They offer shrouds and caskets and will store and transport the body to the cemetery.

Completely green cemeteries are usually some kind of nature preserve. Their burial practices are environmentally friendly, with no tombstones or caskets.

Can I do a Home Burial?

If you live in a rural area you may be allowed to bury a body on your own property if you own the land. Rules and regulations vary from state to state. A few—California, Indiana, and Washington–prohibit home burials. You will need to obtain permits or licenses from your local county or town clerk and follow regulations on the location of the site, the depth of the grave, and any other rules that may apply. Families choose this option because they have a strong connection to their land and it feels more personal.

What Does It All Cost?

If you were to use the full funeral home burial services and add an expensive casket and headstone, you'd be spending tens of thousands of dollars. This is all fine as long as you make those choices when you are in your rational mind and know this is what your loved one would want, and what you or the estate can afford. Here is an average costs of basic funeral home expenses (varying according to coffin choice):

- Burial with embalming, coffin, visitation, and burial service: $6,000 to $13,000.
- Simple cremation in a cardboard coffin and ashes returned in simple container: $1,000 to $3,000.
- Green Burial, which is basically picking up the body, refrigeration, delivery of body to burial site (shrouds and biodegradable coffins are extra): $2,600.
- Direct Cremation: $500 to $1000.

PLANNING THE FUNERAL, MEMORIAL, OR WAKE

A funeral is most often held at a church and is led by a minister or religious advisor. Family members speak; often hymns are sung and pallbearers carry the casket (if there is one) to the hearse.

A memorial or a wake can be anything you want it to be. It should reflect the deceased and the surviving family. There is no right or wrong way to do it. Here are a few that have been in our town:

- Dan's family held a wake at the local Irish pub. They told stories and made toasts to Dan, hefting pints of Dan's favorite brew—Guinness.
- Amy loved daffodils. When she died, her family passed out bags of daffodil bulbs to friends and strangers all over our town with these instructions: Plant them for Amy. Now, every spring, hundreds of daffodils bloom all over Ashland, Oregon in Amy's memory.
- Delores planned her own memorial and was there when it happened. While she was alive, her friends and family were invited over to celebrate her life, look at pictures, tell favorite memories of Delores and sing her favorite songs. When she died, per her request, she was laid out for a day in her home so friends could visit. And when she was cremated, her ashes were divided between her three children.
- Shoshana's family kept her body on dry ice for three days while friends and family brought flowers and covered her with them. They then loaded Shoshana into a station wagon and followed a New Orleans-style marching band around the city park. At the end of the day, Shoshana was taken to the family ranch, where she was buried.

Jahnna

We rented the tiny community center in Ashland, Oregon for Dad's memorial. Friends brought food and I bought champagne and rented glasses from a party supply place. I displayed photos, Dad's artwork, and a book we'd put together of his memories that he called *Ole Daddy Remembers*. There was a guestbook. I introduced my family, told about my Dad's service as a pilot in WW II, and his career in the Air Force. Two of Dad's friends spoke. One read Dad's favorite poem, *High Flight.* We played a video clip of Dad singing a verse from *"I Did It My Way"* at the end of the memorial and drank a toast to Charles Nathan Beecham, who, in the course of his lifetime had many names, including Pinky (because of his red hair), Chuck, Nate, Beech, Charlie, Ole Daddy, and Grandpa.

What Do You Do with the Ashes?

More than 60 percent of people choose cremation over burial. Some choose beautiful urns and keep their loved one's cremains in the home. Many people ask to have their ashes scattered in a specific place:

- Jack took a memorial journey, scattering his wife Susan's ashes in all of the places where they had lived and loved.
- Jahnna's cousin, Ann, requested that her ashes be tossed into the outgoing tide of the Pacific Ocean at sunset to the tune of "Over the Rainbow."
- Ashes can also be pressed into diamonds, sculptures, and pots. They can even be incorporated into paintings.
- In Hawaii, surfers paddle out in the surf with the ashes of their loved one, circle, and toss them into the deep blue makai (ocean) with flower leis.
- Actor Johnny Depp fired the late author Hunter S. Thompson's ashes from a cannon, accompanied by red, white, blue, and green fireworks, to the tune of "Spirit in the Sky."

The Legality of Scattering Ashes

It's probably a good idea to get permission if you are on someone's private property, but otherwise, many suggest a "Don't Ask, Don't Tell" policy.

Should Children Go to Funerals? We have funerals for a reason. They help us honor the dead, say good-bye, and receive support from the community. Children also benefit from them. If your child is old enough to understand and wants to participate, being included may help her share in the support that these gatherings provide. Explain to the child what to expect: People will be sad and may be crying. Children should not be made to feel guilty for not wanting to go.

Jahnna

When my children were five and seven their grandmother Rosie died in another state. There was no official funeral so we created one at our home. The children lit candles in the living room, and then my son played the penny whistle while they walked into the room. They each said what they loved about their grandma and told how much they would miss her. Then we wrote notes to her on a piece of paper and put them in the fire in the fireplace to send the message, now written in smoke, up in the air and out into the world for Rosie to receive.

THE BUSINESS OF DEATH

Important Documents

Be sure to gather in one place, like a portable file box:

- ❑ Trust
- ❑ Will
- ❑ Bank accounts
- ❑ Deeds
- ❑ Tax returns
- ❑ Birth and marriage certificate
- ❑ Business contracts
- ❑ Vehicle registration (cars, boats, trucks, etc.)
- ❑ Loan documents
- ❑ Credit Card Accounts
- ❑ Records needed for tax return

Notify Organizations

Start with: Social Security, Military, retirement accounts, insurance companies, credit card companies, and any subscriptions or services that need to be cancelled. Keep records of who was called, what date, and what was said.

❑ **Social Security Administration:** (800) 772-1213 or www.ssa.gov

They will need a copy of the death certificate. Ask about survivor benefits. There is a $255 death benefit to the surviving spouse.

Note: Social Security will not pay benefits for the month of death. That means if the person died in July, the check received in August (which is payment for July) must be returned. If the payment is by direct deposit, notify the financial institution as soon as possible so it can return any payments received after death.

❑ **Contact Employers** and find out if there is any unpaid salary, pension, unused vacation time, or sick leave.

❑ **Union:** Ask if the deceased had any benefits with the organization.

❑ **Life Insurance:** File a claim and ask what distribution options are available.

- ❑ **Veterans Affairs Office:** (800) 827-1000 or www.va.gov
  - ❑ Contact the Veteran's Administration with the veteran's entry and exit date from service and the discharge papers. These benefits are available:
    - American Flag
    - A grave marker is given to any veteran buried in a recognized cemetery.
    - If the veteran is buried in a National Cemetery, he is entitled to a $450 burial allotment ($150 for plot and $300 for funeral services). If the veteran died because of a service connected disability, he is entitled to $1500 or the cost of the service—whichever is less.

Write an Obituary

The funeral home generally puts a death announcement in the paper for free. If you would like to run an obituary in the newspaper, you'll have to pay for it. (This surprises many people.) Newspapers bill by the word or column inch.

An affordable option would be to have the death announcement direct readers to an online obituary, which would include a picture. You can print this page out and send to alumni organizations, military magazines, company magazines, and other towns where your loved one has lived.

> **Jahnna**
> The Oregonian in Portland, OR costs $100 per column inch, which works out to about 30 words. My dad's obit in two small town papers cost around $350 each.

The Basic Obituary Usually Includes:

- ❑ Full name of the deceased, her age, profession, and where she lived
- ❑ Name of spouse or significant other, children, and grandchildren
- ❑ Time and location of memorial service
- ❑ Significant life events like awards, favorite hobbies, causes she championed, and activities she loved.
- ❑ Name of organization and address where people can send memorial contributions in lieu of flowers.

Order Death Certificates:

A standard amount to order is about ten. You will need them when reporting the death to Social Security, the VA, life insurance, retirement accounts, and the IRS. You may need them to cancel cell phone contracts and memberships. All estates vary, but these organizations will also require them:

- ❑ Trust Accounts
- ❑ Living Trust
- ❑ 401-K
- ❑ IRA
- ❑ Mutual Funds
- ❑ Stocks and Bonds
- ❑ Safety deposit box
- ❑ Health, house, and auto insurance companies

Transfer Ownership or Redeem:

- ❑ Checking and saving accounts
- ❑ Retirement accounts
- ❑ Real estate titles
- ❑ Real estate
- ❑ Automobile titles
- ❑ Stock certificates, bonds, CDs, treasury bills, money market accounts, and IRAs

Jahnna

After Dad died, my brother and I kept certain items of clothing and donated the rest to charity. Dad loved hats. I have his berets, Scottish tams, pith helmet, and military hats in a large Ziploc storage bag. Can't bear to part with those. The adult diapers we donated to hospice. And I gave certain military treasures and model B-17's to his friends. About two months after Dad died, I mailed out cards with an update on mom and a copy of the obituary. It was great because she received a new wave of letters from friends. I think the best thing we did after Dad died was to put all of his papers—death certificates, copies of the obituary, photos of him and social security and VA information into one portable file box. We still find ourselves needing something from that file. Contact the Veteran's Administration with this information with veteran's entry and exit date from service and the discharge papers.

THIRTEEN

HOW TO GO ON LIVING

"It's so curious: one can resist tears and 'behave' very well in the hardest hours of grief. But then someone makes you a friendly sign behind a window, or one notices that a flower that was in bud only yesterday has suddenly blossomed, or a letter slips from a drawer . . . and everything collapses."

—Colette

GRIEF IS NORMAL

Grief is a healing process unique to each individual. You never know what path it will travel or when it will hit—it could be now, six months from now, or even a year. But we all grieve, whether we show it or not.

Jahnna

My mom seemed to be okay for the first six months after Dad died, but suddenly she was exhausted and extremely depressed. She started talking about wanting "death with dignity" and giving me instructions for where to sprinkle her ashes. It wasn't till Katie and I were writing this chapter that I realized what was really going on with Mom—she was finally grieving.

Symptoms of Grief

Grief has physical and mental symptoms as well as emotional ones. It's only natural that such a great loss would manifest itself physically. These symptoms may not appear right away but you may find yourself having stomach problems or insomnia or suddenly being accident-prone. Grief may wash over you when you are walking down the street and your legs nearly give out, or you may find yourself gasping in disbelief months after your loss. You may feel like you are walking around in a fog, unable to think or make decisions of any kind. This is all normal.

Other Symptoms of Grief

Physical

- Deep sighing
- A feeling of heaviness in the chest
- Stomach problems and changes in appetite
- Shortness of breath
- Lowered resistance to illness
- A feeling of tightness in the throat
- Sleeping difficulties
- Fatigue and weakness

Mental

- Difficulty concentrating and focusing
- Feeling aimless and wandering
- Not finishing anything
- Being very forgetful or absentminded

Anger and Guilt

Mourning the loss of a loved one can be multi-layered. You may feel intense anger at the deceased for leaving you alone. Or the last few months may have been a pretty rocky road. Your loved one may have suffered dementia, been mean and angry with you, and you may have wished he would just go.

Guilt can wash over you in waves. Guilt for the last words you said, guilt for having dark thoughts, and guilt for being the one who survived. Again this is all normal. The bottom line is you were there for your loved one.

WHAT'S WRONG WITH ME?

At hospice, Katie checks in with the families after they lose a loved one to see how they are doing. Most of the discussions she has are about grief. Here are some questions she's been asked and her answers:

My mother just died and I can't cry. Is something wrong with me?

It's normal to feel numb during the first month or so. Some people even report feeling "hyper" and are surprised that they aren't feeling bad. It is our body's way of allowing us a break from our strong emotions. This does not mean you are not grieving or feeling sad.

People tell me I shouldn't make big decisions right now. Is this true?

If possible, it is best to put off major decisions, like selling the house, for at least a year, when your judgment is clearer.

It's been four months since my father died and I am feeling worse than ever, crying all the time, and I thought I was doing so well. I feel like I'm going backwards!
It is quite common for grief to feel stronger at around the fourth to the sixth month mark. The numbness that we felt during first few months has worn off and the reality of the loss often hits us like a ton of bricks. You may find yourself feeling very sad or depressed at this time. You want your life to be the same as it was before, but are finally realizing that it can't be.

One minute I'm fine and the next minute I'm sobbing my eyes out. Is this normal?
Yes! Grief is like a rollercoaster ride, with your emotions going up and down and all over the place. It can be very unpredictable. A song, or glancing at an item in the grocery store that your loved one liked, may set you off. You may feel sadness, guilt, fear, anger, or a number of other emotions. Honor your feelings and know that over time they will reside.

I just loss my sister and am comforted by wearing her clothes and even sleeping in her bed. Is this bizarre?
This is normal behavior after losing people we love. The smell of their clothes and sheets or their favorite perfumes can be very comforting. Other behaviors that may seem odd, but are very normal are:

- Searching for or calling out to your loved-one
- Seeing or feeling the presence of the deceased
- Having vivid or "visitation" dreams of the deceased
- Adopting the habits and mannerisms of your loved one
- Being preoccupied with the belongings of the deceased
- Visiting places or people that were important to your loved-one
- Avoiding places that evoke strong memories of the deceased
- Withdrawing from friends and family
- Experiencing manic states of over activity or creativity

Since my husband died five months ago, I don't feel like doing anything or seeing anyone. My friends are worried about me. Should they be?
Your husband's death is still very recent and people oftentimes feel more depressed at five to six months, than right after the loss. Don't push your friends away. Sometimes being around one or two people is easier than being in a large group. You might want to start with a small visit such as a walk or cup of tea with a friend, rather than committing to a long dinner or a larger social situation.

My father left when I was young and we didn't have a very good relationship, but now that he's gone I find myself feeling really sad and even angry. I thought I wouldn't feel much of anything when he died and I'm so confused.
Sometimes we grieve what we didn't have in a relationship, rather than what we lost. As long as someone is alive there is always a chance or hope that things could get better. But when that person dies, the hope vanishes.

When will my grief end?
How long grief lasts varies with each individual. One never stops grieving completely, and our lives will never be the same. Hospice nurse and author Barbara Karnes describes fresh grief as an open wound that is terribly painful, unbearable at times, but with time and care it heals. Yet it leaves a scar that hurts or bothers us from time to time. We adapt to a new normal and gradually the feelings lessen in intensity and frequency.

I couldn't take care of my husband anymore and had to put him in a nursing home a few weeks before he died. I am now feeling incredibly guilty for not keeping him at home.
After a death most of us feel guilt or regret because we didn't do or say something we should have, or we did say or do something we wish we hadn't. Just remember you did the best you could at the time with the information and coping skills that you had. Though it is normal to feel some guilt and have regrets, we also need to forgive ourselves and let it go. If you your guilt is prolonged and causing you emotional distress, talk with a grief counselor.

When should I clean out my loved-one's closet?
You will know when the time is right. I'd advise waiting a few months or so to remove or throw away these items. Some people regret getting rid of things so quickly. Some find comfort in having the loved one's things around for a while. Others feel all right with cleaning out closets and drawers right away and have no regrets at all. Again, grief is very individual. You need to do what feels right for you.

The holidays are coming and I am feeling anxious that I won't be able to handle them. What should I do?
Talk with your family about your feelings because they are probably feeling the same way. This may be a time when you want extra support from friends or a support group. Holidays, anniversaries, and birthdays can be difficult. You may want to come up with a plan for how to handle these days, such

as keeping the activities simple this year. Try changing the routine and creating a ritual to honor the departed: have a toast, light a candle, and share memories and pictures.

I feel so tired and forgetful all the time. Could this be from grief?
Absolutely! Remember, grief has physical and mental symptoms as well as emotional ones. Feeling exhausted is one of the more common complaints.

HOW DO I GET THROUGH MY GRIEF?

- Start by being kind to yourself. Take care of your health. Eat well and get enough sleep. Exercise can help release feelings of sadness and tension. Take the time you need to reflect on your loss.
- Allow yourself to talk about your loss with friends, counselors or in support groups. Cry about your loss. Tears do not mean you are weak or losing control.
- Write about your feelings of grief. Or create a journal of great memories with the deceased. It doesn't have to be a full-blown book, just snippets of funny, wonderful, meaningful exchanges. A description of your favorite adventures you shared, etc.
- Don't feel guilty for having good days or enjoying yourself. You know your loved one would have wanted you to be happy and go on living a full life.
- If you feel like you're wandering through the days, give yourself a schedule and try to stick with it. Get up at the same time, eat your meals on time and go to bed at the same time. The schedule should include exercise, even if it is a 15-minute walk around the neighborhood or a park.
- Create special rituals for holidays and birthdays that will celebrate your loved one. Light candles, look at photo albums, visit the grave with flowers, or play music and dance.
- Winston Churchill said, "If you're going through hell, keep going." Keep going forward and eventually that pain will not necessarily pass, but it will change into something you will be able to live with.

STUCK IN GRIEF: WHEN GRIEF IS COMPLICATED

When you are locked into grief, it can cause a deep depression that makes it difficult to do anything. When this overwhelming grief lasts well beyond six months, it is often called "complicated grief." Well-meaning family and friends might tell you to get over it, get on with life, think of your kids, just snap out of it, and look at the beauty that's all around you. What they don't understand is that you can't just turn it off—if you could, you would have a long time ago. Your body and your mind are locked in a deep depression. This depression can affect your own health and lead to high blood pressure, strokes, drug and alcohol abuse and even suicide. You don't have to forget your loved one or "just get over" the loss. But you can find ways to live with the loss and look forward to the future.

Risk Factors for Complicated Grief:

- A traumatic death, loss of a young spouse, or loss of a child
- Major life stresses i.e.: financial or health problems
- History of mental illness, especially depression and suicide attempts
- Lack of support systems and isolation
- A dysfunctional or overly dependent relationship with the deceased
- History of alcohol or drug abuse

Signs and Symptoms of Complicated Grief:

- Constant focus on the loss and your loved one
- Intense and almost constant longing for the deceased
- Difficulty accepting the death
- Trouble carrying out normal activities
- Inability to enjoy life
- Withdrawing from social activities
- Lack of trust in others
- Severing friendships
- Agitation, irritability, and guilt
- Feeling a bitterness that colors everything
- Fear of going out, or engaging in activities
- Feeling that life holds no meaning
- Strong thoughts of suicide
- Abusing alcohol or drugs

Katie

Several months after my sister, Dani, died, I started taking an antidepressant. I did not want to at first, thinking my depression was "normal" and I wasn't one of those people that needed drugs. But my doctor explained it like this, "If you were a diabetic and needed insulin, you would take it, right? Well right now you are suffering from a mood disorder and your brain needs more of a certain neurotransmitter to help correct this."

Not until I started taking the antidepressant, did I realize just how depressed I had been. As the months went by after my sister died, I felt myself being pulled down into a deeper and deeper hole. I found it getting harder and harder to drag myself out of bed in the morning and care for my two young children. I had no patience with them. I was worried about the effect of my depression on them, especially after my 3-year-old son walked in on me screaming in my room one day.

The anti-depressant helped pull me out of that dark hole. I still grieved and felt all of my emotions, but they weren't crippling me anymore. I could actually play and laugh again.

What to Do:

Like PTSD and deep depression, complicated grief really requires the help of a health care professional. The therapist may recommend antidepressants combined with talk-therapy. You may think the idea of taking drugs or talking to a therapist is something you would never ever do, but it can help you get unstuck. Anti-depressants work by keeping the good chemicals and neurotransmitters in the brain longer. These brain chemicals will lift your mood and decrease the severity of your depression. Once you feel physically better, you may be open to talking through your grief.

Talk therapy provides tools for altering your thinking and a place to practice healthy thought habits. Support groups are good for sharing your burden with others and finding new strategies for helping yourself loosen the grip that pain has on your life.

> ***Grief is like a wound. At first, it's open, bleeding, raw, and terribly painful. In time that wound begins to heal.***
> ***It heals from the inside out. The pain begins to fade and eventually a scar is formed . . .***
> ***There will always be a scar.***
> ***We will never be the same again.***
>
> —Barbara Karnes

HOW DO I HELP MY CHILDREN GRIEVE?

- Be sure to set aside time to talk to your children, as soon as possible after the death. Share and explain your emotions and don't be afraid to cry in front of them. This allows them to share their grief with you.
- Use correct terms, telling your children that their loved one has "died" or is "dead." Terms like "he went to sleep" or "she has gone to heaven" may cause misunderstanding and more fear later on.
- Use appropriate terms for your child's age and don't over explain. Your child will ask more questions as she needs to, even months or years later, as she matures and is able to understand more. Let her guide the way.
- Let your children be a part of the funeral or service. Show them the casket or ashes. Let them be involved in a ritual such as placing a photo, note or flower in the casket or with the body before cremation.
- Help your children create a memorial, such as a special garden or alter, a memory box or book to honor the deceased.
- Create ways for the children to cope with their grief writing letters to the deceased and reading them out loud or punching a pillow and yelling if they are angry.
- Alert the teacher or school counselor of your child's loss.
- Celebrate the memory of your loved one at birthdays and holidays. Look at photo albums; toast their memory with sparkling cider, share memories or songs.
- Read age appropriate books about grief to your children. See Suggested Reading (pg. 189).

A Child's Symptoms of Grief

Watch out for behavioral and emotional changes at school as well as at home. Some of these might include:

- Bad dreams
- Complaints of stomach aches
- Bed-wetting and other regressive behaviors
- Irritability or moodiness
- Increased clingingness
- Fear of the dark
- Aggressive behavior
- Drop in grades

Katie

A young boy lost his dad and he was very angry and acting out. His mother got him a plastic bat to swing at the tree and it really helped him let go of some of his anger. Then a volunteer sewed him a pillow out of his dad's old flannel shirt that he could hug. His mom also took him to a children's support group.

These behaviors usually resolve on their own, but if they persist or get worse, you may want to seek out professional help through a counselor. Look into support groups that have specialized groups for children of different ages. It has been shown that children helping children can be very beneficial. Mostly, try to spend more time with your child—listening, comforting, and encouraging her expression of feelings.

For help finding children support groups see Online Resources (pg. 185).

Seize the moments of happiness, love and be loved!
That is the only reality in the world, all else is folly.

—Leo Tolstoy

GONE FROM SIGHT

I am standing upon the seashore.
A ship at my side spreads her white
sails to the morning breeze
and starts for the blue ocean.
She is an object of beauty and strength.
I stand and watch her until at last she
hangs like a speck of white cloud
just where the sea and sky come down
to mingle with each other.

Then someone at my side says,
"There she's gone!"
Gone where?
Gone from my sight . . . that is all.

She is just as large in mast and hull
and spar as she was when she left my side.
And just as able to bear her load of
living freight to the place of destination.
Her diminished size is in me, not in her.

And just at the moment
when someone at my side says,
"There, she is gone!"
There are other eyes watching her coming
and other voices ready to take up the
glad shout,
"Here she comes!"

—Henry Van Dyke (1852-1933)

Katie

While writing this book with Jahnna, memories of all the patients and families that I have cared for over the years flooded my mind. What struck me most was the enormous courage and strength these families showed in their final acts of love. Living with dying is hard work, on so many levels. But never forget that being present, day after day, is the best gift you can offer your loved one. And this gift works both ways. So many families have told me that they wouldn't have traded those last months, weeks, and days with their loved ones for anything.

Jahnna

There is the practical journey that caregivers and the dying take and the emotional journey. My dad Charlie was a very funny man who was instantly loved by everyone he met. What most people didn't know was my dad had mild dementia for about the last five years before he died, which translated into him being the world's cutest guy in public and the grumpy, stubborn, irritable man that his family dealt with at home. Not all the time, mind you, but enough to make it unpleasant pretty often. He was particularly mad at me—maybe because I saw the dementia.

But when he was dying, I was there caring for him, working with the nurses to make sure his meds were right, reading all the pamphlets and asking questions of Katie. Dad's world got continually smaller. He no longer was able to participate in Kiwanis or sing in the Meadowlarks choir. Entertaining visitors and talking on the phone was just too taxing. His world was really my mom, my husband, hospice, and me.

Caregiving was often stressful and crazy-making, but I'm so very grateful that I was able to be there to help him through those last months, days, hours, and minutes of life. Toward the end, he thanked me every single day and told me how much he loved me. And one of the last things he did was smile at me from his bed and murmur, "My daughter . . ."

I have Katie to thank for his good death. I knew Katie's twenty-five years of wisdom needed to be in a book. Now it is. We hope it will help other daughters, sons, husbands and wives assist their loved ones in having the best final journey possible.

Part Four

RESOURCE GUIDE

Medical Terminology and Abbreviations

A

ABD: abdomen.

acupuncture: the insertion of small needles into specific points on the body in which energy is believed to be blocked. It can help relieve symptoms such as pain, anxiety, and fluid build-up.

acute: a sharp rise; very active, as in the case of pain.

adjuvant: "in addition to" initial treatment. Adjuvant medications are "helper" medications, usually used in addition to other meds.

ADL: activities of daily living such as dressing, bathing, and feeding oneself.

ALS: amyotrophic lateral sclerosis, or Lou Gehrig's disease, is a neurodegenerative disease affecting the nerve cells of the brain and spinal cord, leading to progressive paralysis of voluntary muscles.

antiemetic: drug that treats nausea and vomiting.

anuric: not producing urine.

aphasia: unable to speak or communicate, often caused by a stroke.

apnea: a pause or stop in breathing.

apneic breathing: a pattern of breathing that involves long pauses in breathing, sometimes for up to a minute. It is commonly seen in people who are close to death.

ASA: acetylsalicylic acid, or aspirin.

ascites: accumulation of fluid in the abdomen.

ATC: around the clock.

B

BID: (Latin bis in die) twice a day. Usually seen on a prescription.

BM: bowel movement.

bolus: an extra dose of pain medication, usually given intravenously for swift response to pain.

bone mets: cancer that has traveled into the bones from another part of the body.

BP: blood pressure.

breakthrough pain: a spike or increase in pain, even though the patient is on a routine dose of pain medication, usually requiring additional medication.

BSC: bedside commode is a portable toilet or "potty-chair" that can be used when the patient is unable to get to the bathroom.

C

CA: cancer.

CAD: coronary artery disease.

Candida: a yeast-like infection

carcinoma: a type of cancer that occurs in the tissue that lines or covers organs and glands like breast, stomach, pancreas, uterus.

CBC: complete blood count.

CC (or ml): cubic centimeter, a measure of volume.

C Diff: clostridium difficile is bacteria that can cause diarrhea, especially in hospitalized elderly patients, and people who have been taking antibiotics.

central line: a thin plastic tube surgically placed into a large blood vessel near the heart. It is used for drawing blood and giving IV medications/fluids.

Cheyne-Stokes: irregular breathing pattern that alternates between shallow breaths to deep, rapid breathing with periods of apnea in between.

CHF: congestive heart failure.

CO2: carbon dioxide.

COPD: chronic obstructive pulmonary disease; emphysema.

CPR: cardiopulmonary resuscitation is a series of heart compressions and rescue breathing performed on a person to revive him after his heart and breathing have stopped.

CT or CAT Scan: multi-series of X-rays that give a cross-section view of the body. It provides more detailed information then an X–ray and is used most for diagnostic purposes.

CVA: cerebral vascular accident; stroke.

D—E

diuretic: medication that removes unwanted fluid from areas such as lungs and legs, by increasing urine output.

Dx: diagnosis

DME: durable medical equipment such as wheelchairs, hospital beds, commodes, or oxygen.

DNR: do not resuscitate; an order or form signed by a doctor so that CPR is not performed if a person's heart and breathing have stopped.

dysphagia: difficulty swallowing.

dyspnea: difficulty breathing.

edema: the swelling or accumulation of fluid in a part of the body.

electric lift chair: a recliner that can lift a person to a standing position.

F—G

Foley catheter: tube inserted into the bladder to drain urine.

FX: fracture.

fracture pan: a small, wedge-shaped bedpan used for patients that cannot sit up or use a standard bedpan.

gait belt: canvas belt placed around the patient's waist that is used to guide and support him when being transferred and walking.

GI: gastrointestinal

G-tube: gastric tube that is surgically placed into the stomach through the abdominal wall. It is used for giving liquid nutrition and medications.

H—J

Hoyer lift: a hydraulic lift that uses a sling to lift the patient and transfer him to bed or a chair.

H&P: history and physical.

HS: at night; hour of sleep.

HX: history.

hypoxia: lack of oxygen; low oxygen in the blood.

IM: intramuscular, as in giving an IM injection.

incontinent inability to retain urine or stool due to loss of sphincter control, or due to cerebral/spinal damage.

IV: intravenous; meds or fluid given into the vein.

jaundice: yellowish coloring of the skin and whites of the eyes, from the accumulation of too much bilirubin in the blood.

K—M

lymphatic system: a network of lymphatic vessels that carry fluid (lymph fluid), nutrients, and waste material between the body tissues and the bloodstream. It helps the body fight infection.

MRI: magnetic resonance imagery; a more powerful and exact scan than the CT.

metastasis/mets: the spread of cancer cells from the original tumor through the blood and lymphatic system to another part of the body.

Mg: milligrams; a measure of weight used for dosing medications.

Ml (or cc): milliliter; measure of volume.

MRSA: methicillin-resistant staphylococcus aureus is a bacteria that's become resistant to many antibiotics and is difficult to treat.

N—O

N/V: nausea/vomiting.

Ng Tube: a nasogastric tube that is inserted through the nose into the stomach for feeding or suctioning.

No Code: same as a DNR—do not resuscitate.

NPO: (Latin nil per os) nothing by mouth.

NSAID: non-steroidal anti-inflammatory drug like ibuprofen or aspirin.

NTG: nitroglycerin is a med used for chest pain.

O2: oxygen.

OTC: over the counter; non-prescription drugs.

P—Q

palliative sedation: when a patient who is close to dying is administered a sedating drug and is allowed to sleep until the death occurs. This is for patients who are suffering from uncontrollable symptoms.

paracentesis: needle inserted into the abdominal cavity to remove fluid.

PO: (Latin per os) by mouth

PC/ Port-A-Cath: surgically implanted chamber under the skin in the upper chest with access to a major artery or vein, used for IV therapy.

PR: per rectum.

PRN: (Latin pro re nata) use as needed.

QD: (Latin quaque die) once a day; every day.

QID: (Latin quater in die) 4 times a day.

R—T

RBC: red blood count

reflexology: the practice of applying pressure to specific points in the hands and feet using special thumb, finger, and hand techniques. The belief is that certain areas in the hands and feet correspond to an organ or area of the body, and this practice can provide pain relief and other symptom relief.

Rx: prescription medicine

SOB: shortness of breath

somatic pain: general pain that can be easily identified, like pain from stubbing a toe or breaking an arm. It is often described as sharp, stabbing, throbbing, or aching.

SSRI: selective serotonin re-uptake inhibitors are antidepressants used to treat major depression and anxiety.

sub-q: subcutaneous; beneath the skin.

sub-q pump: a small subcutaneous catheter inserted under the skin to deliver medication by a programmed pump, usually for pain.

Sx: symptom.

thoracentesis: a needle is inserted into the space around the lung to remove fluid.

TIA: transient ischemic attack—a mini-stroke.

TID: 3 times a day.

trapeze: a large metal triangle that is hung from a bar secured over a hospital bed, that a patient can hold onto for lifting and positioning herself.

Tx: treatment.

U—Z

URI: upper respiratory infection.

UTI: urinary tract infection.

visceral pain: organ pain; often described as cramping or spasms in the liver, intestines, stomach, and other organs. The pain often radiates to other parts of the abdomen or back, and can feel like a tight band around the person's midsection.

void: to evacuate the bowels or bladder.

WBC: white blood count.

These medications have been mentioned in our book and are commonly used in the care of critically ill patients. We've listed the generic name and the well-known brand name in alphabetical order.

A

Acetaminophen (Tylenol): an OTC analgesic used for minor aches and pains, and to reduce fever.

Acyclovir (Zovirax): treats viral infections, including shingles, herpes, and chicken-pox. Can be given orally, IV, or as an ointment.

Advil (Ibuprofen): treats mild to moderate pain and fever; it is a non-steroidal anti-inflammatory, or NSAID.

Afrin: a nasal decongestant spray that can sometimes help with nosebleeds.

Aleve (Naproxen): treats mild to moderate pain and fever; it is a NSAID that is taken every 12 hours.

Aspirin (ASA): used for mild to moderate pain and fever, and also taken to reduce heart attack and stroke. Sometimes given immediately after a heart attack or stroke to prevent worsening or recurrence of symptoms.

Atarax (Hydroxyzine,Vistaril): an antihistamine used to treat anxiety, nausea, vomiting, allergies, and skin conditions such as rashes, hives, and itching.

Ativan (Lorazepam): treats anxiety and insomnia, can also help nausea. Used in end-of-life care for shortness of breath and restlessness. Crush and mix with a few drops of water and place under the tongue.

Atropine: used to treat spasmodic pain of the gastrointestinal, stomach, and biliary tract. It is also used to drecrease throat secretions.

B

Baclofen (Lioresal): is an oral and injectable muscle relaxant used to treat painful spasms of the skeletal muscles due to multiple sclerosis, cerebral palsy, and diseases or injuries to the spinal cord or brain.

Belladona and Opium Suppositories (referred to as a "B&O"): used rectally and vaginally to treat spasmodic pain of the urinary tract and pelvic floor.

Benadryl (Diphenhydramine): an over-the-counter antihistamine commonly used for allergies; also can help with itching and insomnia.

C

Canasol: synthetic marijuana in pill form, prescribed by a doctor.

Celexa (Citalopram): a SSRI antidepressant, mostly used for depression but can help with anxiety disorders as well.

Colace (Docusate sodium): stool softener.

Compazine (Prochlorperazine): treats nausea and vomiting. It can be given by mouth, rectally, or by IV.

Coumadin (Warfarin): an anticoagulant, or blood thinner, that prevents new clots from forming and existing ones from getting worse. Blood tests are routinely taken to make sure the dose is right.

D

Decadron (Dexamethasone): a potent steroid and powerful anti-inflammatory used to treat pain and symptoms in many diseases such as in brain tumors, bone pain from cancer, and multiple myeloma at the end of life. Can also help with nausea and vomiting, and can boost appetite and fight fatigue.

Depakote (Valproic acid): an anticonvulsant that can be used for treating mood disorders such as bipolar, and those found in Alzheimer's disease.

Diflucan (Fluconazole): an antifungal drug used to treat stubborn thrush infections when mycostatin swish-and-swallow or a topical doesn't work.

Dilantin (Phenytoin): anti-seizure drug

Dilaudid (Hydromorphone): a narcotic analgesic used for moderate to severe pain. It is a semi-synthetic derivative of morphine, and sometimes has fewer side effects than morphine.

Ditropan (Oxybutynin): used to treat bladder spasms, primarily in end of life care, to control spasms caused by indwelling urinary catheters.

Dulcolax (Bisacodyl): a stimulant laxative used for constipation. It comes in pills, rectal suppositories, and enemas; sold over-the-counter.

Duragesic patch (Fentanyl): a synthetic opioid patch placed on the skin and changed every 3 days. It provides relief for severe chronic pain.

E—F

Elavil (Amitriptyline): a tricyclic antidepressant used for neuropathic pain and insomnia, and may help with itching.

Famvir (Famciclovir): antiviral drug that is used to treat shingles and other herpes infections.

Flagyl (Metronidazole) is an antibiotic used to treat C-diff. In powder form it reduces the smell in wounds.

Flomax (Tamsulosin) relaxes the muscles in the prostate and bladder neck, making it easier for men to urinate.

G—H

Guaifenesin syrup: narcotic cough syrup that loosens secretions.

Haldol (Haloperidol): an anti-psychotic used for severe agitation, especially for those patients with dementia or Alzheimer's. It can also help treat severe nausea and vomiting, and intractable hiccups.

I—J

Ibuprofen (Advil): treats mild to moderate pain and fever; it is a nonsteroidal anti-inflammatory or NSAID.

Imodium: an over-the-counter drug used to treat and control diarrhea.

Inapsine (Droperidol): used in IM or IV form to control severe nausea and vomiting, especially in patients with bowel obstructions. It also helps with anxiety and can be sedating.

Indocin (Indomethacin): a prescription NSAID used for mild to moderate pain.

K—L

Keppra (Levetiracetam): anti-seizure drug

Klonopin (Clonazepam): an anti-seizure, anti-anxiety drug that can be used for anxiety, panic attacks, and mood disorders.

Lactulose: a syrup-like medication used for constipation, and to reduce ammonia in the body of patients with liver disease.

Lasix (Furosemide): a diuretic (water pill) used to pull fluid out of spaces in the body and the extremities. The patient pees it out. It is also used to relieve shortness of breath in heart failure.

Levsin (Hyoscyamine): used to control spasmodic pain in the GI tract. It can also reduce salivary secretions.

Lidocaine (Xylocaine): in gel or patch form it is used to numb tissue in a certain area.

Lortab elixir: liquid form of Vicodin (acetaminophen and hydrocodone), which is a pain reliever.

M—N

Marinol: the synthetic form of marijuana (THC) that is legal when prescribed by a doctor. It is used for nausea and vomiting, and as an appetite stimulant.

Methadone: a synthetic opioid used for moderate to severe pain. May be more effective than other opioids for neuropathic pain, and can be dosed less frequently.

Miconazole: antifungal over-the-counter medication used for yeast infections.

Miralax: a medication in powder form that is mixed with water or juice to treat constipation.

Milk of Magnesia (MOM): a liquid medication used for constipation and as an antacid.

Morphine: considered the gold standard of pain medications, it is a narcotic painkiller used frequently in end-of-life care. It is used for moderate to severe pain and comes in a fast-acting pill, liquid form, or in a time-released pill. It can also be given IV or SC by a pump. It is very effective in relieving shortness of breath found with diseases such as congestive heart failure and COPD. Also used to treat angina (heart pain).

Neurontin (Gabapentin): originally developed for seizures, it is also used to treat neuropathic pain.

Nitroglycerin (Nitro, NG): used to treat angina or heart pain by dilating the blood vessels in the heart. It can be taken as a small pill under the tongue, a mouth spray, or a patch on the skin.

Norco: Vicodin, which is an opioid narcotic analgesic drug combined with Tylenol, used to treat moderate pain.

Nystatin: an antifungal medication that comes in a swish-and-swallow suspension for thrush and esophageal yeast, as well as a cream and powder form for other areas of the body.

O—P

Oxycodone: a semi-synthetic opioid painkiller used to treat moderate to severe pain.

Oxycontin: a time-released form of oxycodone that is taken every 8-12 hours. (It should not be crushed.)

Pamelor (Nortriptyline): a tricyclic antidepressant, also used to treat nerve pain. It has less sedating effects than elavil (amitriptyline).

Paxil (Paroxetine): an SSRI (selective serotonin reuptake inhibitor) antidepressant also used for panic attacks and anxiety disorders.

Percocet (Oxycodone and Acetaminophen): an opioid analgesic used for moderate to moderately severe pain.

Phenobarbital: a barbiturate used for seizures and sometimes, at the end-of-life, for sedation if agitation cannot be controlled by other means. It can be given orally or rectally.

Prednisone: a steroid used to reduce inflammation in the lungs of patients with COPD. Also an anticancer drug used in people with leukemia, lymphoma, and multiple myeloma.

Prevacid (Lansoprazole): used for heartburn by reducing the production of acid in the stomach.

Prilosec (Omeprazole): used for heartburn by reducing production of acid in the stomach.

Pyridium (Phenazopyridine): an analgesic that is used to relieve pain, burning, and discomfort from urinary tract infections. It is not an antibiotic, so will not treat the infection itself. It also turns the urine dark orange, so don't be alarmed.

Q—R

Reglan (Metoclopramide): is normally used to treat heartburn, but in end of life care it is used for nausea and vomiting.

Remeron (Mirtazapine): antidepressant used for sleep.

Risperdal (Risperidone): an anti-psychotic used mostly in patients with severe agitation and mood disorders.

Ritalin (Methylphenidate): a stimulant commonly used for ADHD that can be effective in treating opioid-induced fatigue and lethargy.

Robinul (Glycopyrronium bromide): used to decrease secretions in the mouth and throat.

S

Sarna: a steroid-free anti-itch lotion.

Scopolamine ("Scop-patch"): a small patch placed behind the ear that helps dry up secretions in the throat, and can also relieve spasms in the GI and biliary tracts.

Senna: a laxative used to treat constipation.

Senokot-S: combination of senna and colace, to treat constipation.

Seroquel (Quetiapine): an anti-psychotic used for extreme mood disorders and agitation in end of life care, mostly in patients with dementia and/or bipolar symptoms.

Soma (Carisoprodol): a muscle relaxant used for pain, muscle stiffness, and muscle spasms.

T

Tegretol (Carbamazepine): an anti-seizure, mood-stabilizing drug used to treat nerve pain.

Thorazine (Chlorpromazine): an anti-psychotic, used at times in end of life care for severe air hunger (shortness of breath) and severe hiccups. It also helps with severe nausea and vomiting, and agitation.

Tofranil (Imipramine): an antidepressant that may help with itching.

Trazodone (Oleptro, Desyrel): an antidepressant used as a sleeping aid.

Tylenol (Acetaminophen): an over-the-counter analgesic, used for minor aches and pains, and to reduce fever.

U—V

Ultram (Tramadol): an opioid analgesic, used to treat moderate to moderately severe pain.

Valium (Diazepam): used to treat anxiety, seizures, and muscle spasms.

Versed (Midazolam): used very rarely in end of life care, when a patient chooses to be sedated (palliative sedation) in the final days of life. This drug is given IV or SC by a pump. Also in nasal spray form, for seizures and bleeding out (to sedate patient).

Vicodin (Hydrocodone and Acetaminophen): an opioid narcotic analgesic drug combined with Tylenol, used to treat moderate pain.

Vicoprofen (Hydrocodone and Ibuprofen): an opioid narcotic analgesic drug combined with Advil, used to treat moderate pain.

Vistaril (hydroxyzine): antihistamine used to treat itching and anxiety.

X—Z

Xanax (Alprazolam): used for anxiety, insomnia, and shortness of breath.

Zantac (Ranitidine): treats and prevents heartburn.

Zofran (Ondansetron): a very effective drug used for nausea and vomiting.

Zoloft (Sertraline): a SSRI antidepressant used also for obsessive-compulsive disorder, panic, and anxiety disorders.

THE BEST MEDS FOR THE BEST PAIN CONTROL

The World Health Organization created a pain ladder for determining the right medication for different levels of pain. You don't want to leap to morphine the minute someone starts having pain. Sometimes someone with mild to moderate pain does quite well with a couple of Tylenol a day. As pain worsens, with the advice of a nurse or doctor, you can move up the pain ladder.

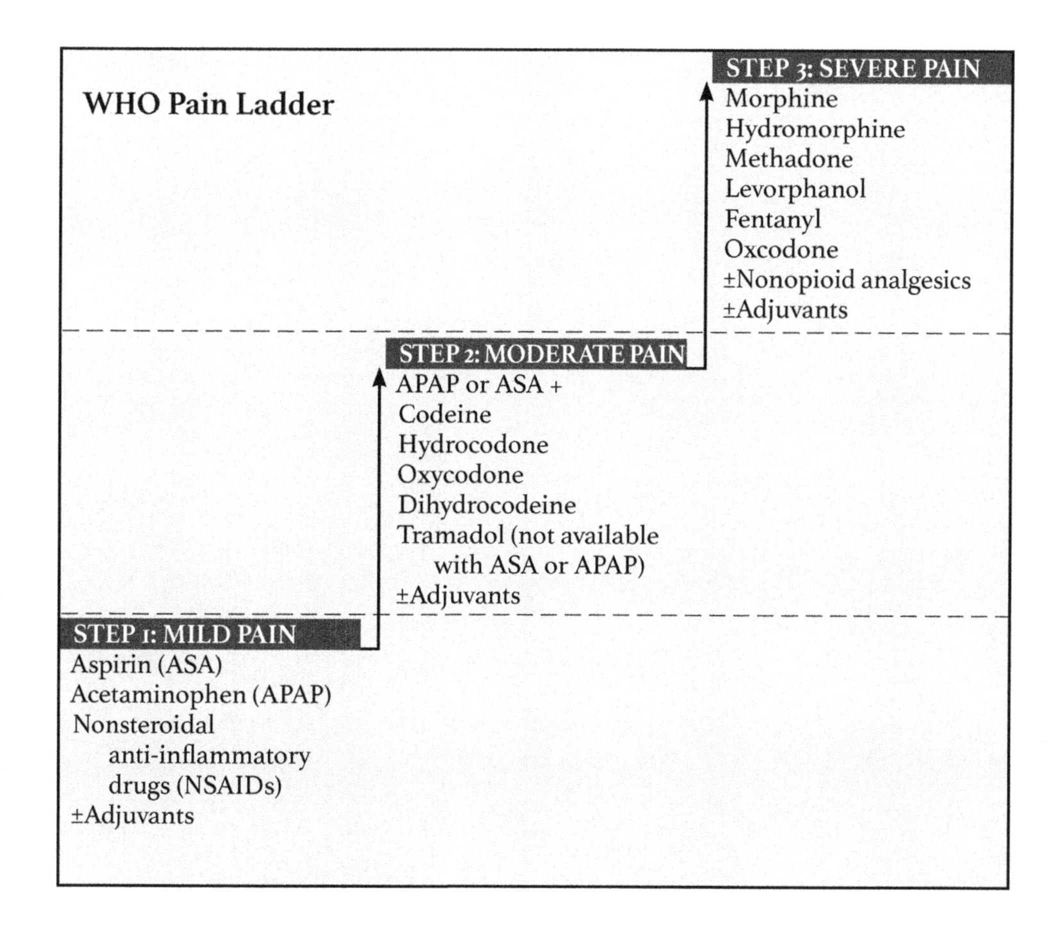

EVERPLANS is a secure digital archive of everything your loved ones will need should something happen to you. It includes trusts, insurance policies, accounts and passwords, health and medical information, final wishes, advanced directives and DNRs. The company's motto is "Leave a legacy, not a mess."

www.everplans.com

THE BIG BOOK OF EVERYTHING is a notebook of forms that covers everything anyone could possibly need to know about you. The idea is to fill it out and keep it current—bank accounts, safe deposit box, storage bin and location of key, health insurance, life insurance, IRAs, trust information, wills, online accounts, passwords, property tax information, subscriptions, pre-paid funeral information, obituary, etc. This printable book is free and was put together by Erik A. Dewey.

www.erikdewey.com/bigbook.htm

LAW DEPOT—free legal forms including wills, power of attorney, durable power of attorney forms, trusts, and contracts.

www.Lawdepot.com

ADVANCE DIRECTIVES

CARINGINFO provides free advance directives and instructions for each state that can be opened as a PDF file and printed.

www.caringinfo.org

FIVE WISHES—The Five Wishes Advance Directive form lets your loved ones know your health care choices if you are too sick to make them. The whole document can be downloaded and filled out at the website:

www.agingwithdignity.org

THE CONVERSATION PROJECT is a website dedicated to helping people talk about their wishes for end of life care. It began in 2010, when Ellen Goodman and a group of colleagues and concerned media, clergy, and medical professionals gathered to share stories of "good deaths" and "bad deaths" within their own circle of loved ones. The site offers a resource center and a conversation starter kit to help you begin.

www.Converstaionproject.org

MY GIFT OF GRACE is a conversation game. In the $24.95 game box, you'll find an instruction sheet, 47 question cards, and 24 thank you chips. Questions in the game cover a wide variety of topics about living and dying well, with all the players having a chance to share their answers to the same question. The website offers tips for going from starting the conversation to taking action.

www.mygiftofgrace.com

ALZHEIMER'S DISEASE AND DEMENTIA ADVANCE DIRECTIVE can be found at the Alzheimer's website.

www.alz.org

CAREGIVER SUPPORT

THE ALZHEIMER'S ASSOCIATION will provide contact information about support groups for caregivers of sufferers of Alzheimer's disease and related disorders.

1-800-272-3900
www.alz.org

AMERICAN ASSOCIATION OF RETIRED PERSONS (AARP) Go to "Caregiving" on their website to find their Caregiving Resource Center, Care Provider Locator and a Long Term Care calculator. You don't need to be a retired person to find valuable information on this site.

www.aarp.org/home-family/caregiving

CARING BRIDGE is a website that helps family and friends keep up to date with their loved one's health journey. It limits the need for answering the same questions over and over again. News is posted on the website and messages can be left.

www.Caringbridge.org

CARING CONNECTIONS provides resources and valuable information on end of life care, who pays for hospice, the business of dying, handling pain, grief and loss.

www.Caringinfo.org

ELDERCARE LOCATOR is a free national directory to help you identify aging services in your community including transportation, housing options, home health services, home delivered meals, adult day care, respite services, and legal assistance.

1-800-677-116 (Monday through Friday 9 a.m. to 8 p.m. EST)
www.eldercare.gov

FAITH IN ACTION is a network of organizations that help chronically ill, elderly, and disabled persons. Volunteers shop, visit, read aloud to patients, and take them to appointments.

www.fiavolunteers.org

THE FAMILY CAREGIVER ALLIANCE is based in San Francisco and is a self-described public voice for caregivers. The FCA website includes state by state listings of resources for caregivers, how to find and create support groups, caregiving for dementia, caregiving for a veteran, newsletters, and other websites for families who are caring for loved ones with chronic or disabling health conditions.

1-800-445-8106
www.caregiver.org

THE WELL SPOUSE FOUNDATION wants you to know you are not alone. They offer support and address the needs of spouses who are caring for a chronically ill and/or disabled spouse/partner. The organization publishes a newsletter, facilitates a mentor program, and coordinates a national network of support groups.

1-800-838-0879
www.wellspouse.org

FINDING A CARE MANAGER

AGING LIFE CARE ASSOCIATION—Though most clients are seniors who need ongoing care management, managers work with patients of all ages. They have an easy-to-use finder for a care manager in your area.

www.aginglifecare.org

LONGTERM CARE

LONGTERMCARE.GOV—This site addresses longterm care, how to find ways to pay for it, like using life insurance to fund the care. It also gives state specific information about what you can do to pay for care.

www.longtermcare.gov

MEDICARE COVERAGE OF SKILLED NURSING FACILITY CARE is a pamphlet published by the Centers for Medicare and Medicaid Services. It explains what's covered and where to get answers to your questions.

1-800-633-4227—ask for publication #10153
www.medicare.gov—click on Publications.

VETERAN'S ADMINISTRATION—Call the VA to find out if your veteran is eligible for free or low-cost nursing home care.

1-800-827-1000
www.va.gov

HOSPICE

NATIONAL HOSPICE AND PALLIATIVE CARE ORGANIZATION will tell you everything you need to know about hospice and who to call in your area.

(703) 837-1500
www.NHPCO.org

NATIONAL HOSPICE FOUNDATION helps you find a hospice program in your area, lists programs and websites you can access for support, and gives you information about pain control.

www.nationalhospicefoundation.org

RIGHT TO DIE OPTION

DEATH WITH DIGNITY NATIONAL CENTER gives Information on U.S. polling, state legislation, the Oregon Death with Dignity Act, and the case of Oregon v. Ashcroft. Find out the laws and how to access them on this site.

www.deathwithdignity.org

FINAL EXIT by Derek Humphrey (1991) is a New York Times best-selling book that examines "The practicalities of self deliverance and assisted suicide for the dying."

FINAL EXIT NETWORK supports the human right to a death with dignity. It is a great resource site that includes information on the World Federation of Right to Die Societies, the World Federation Conference, the death with dignity movement, right to self-determination, support groups, and more.

(866) 654-9156
www.finalexitnetwork.org

FINDING A FUNERAL HOME

FUNERALHOMES.COM—This website will help you find a listing of funeral homes in your area and their contact numbers.

www.FuneralHomes.com

GRIEF SUPPORT

GRIEF SHARE is a website that helps you find grief support groups that are meeting in your area.

www.griefshare.org

GRIEFNET provides online support for those dealing with grief and loss issues.

www.griefnet.org

THE COMPASSIONATE FRIENDS (TCF) provides grief support for parents after the death of a child.

www.compassionatefriends.org

THE DOUGY CENTER is the national center for grieving children and families

www.dougy.org

PODCASTS

ALZHEIMERS SPEAKS with Lori La Bey
Alzheimer's Speaks Radio gives voice to those afflicted with memory loss and their care partners. The goal is to raise awareness, give hope, and share the real everyday life of living with dementia.

www.blogtalkradio.com/alzheimersspeaks

END OF LIFE UNIVERSITY with Karen Wyatt provides online support for those dealing with grief and loss issues.
Dr. Wyatt, a hospice physician and author of *What Really Matters,* interviews experts on all aspects of the end-of-life including: caring for the dying, conscious dying, caregiver support, grief and loss, and afterlife.

https://eoluniversity.com

GOOD GRIEF with Cheryl Jones
On Good Grief, Cheryl Jones talks with people about the losses that define our lives. Grief can teach you what your strengths are and ignite your courage. It can heighten what is important to you and help you let go of what is not.

https://www.stitcher.com/podcast/voice-america/good-grief

HEART OF HOSPICE with Helen Bauer, RN and Jerry Fenter, Chaplain
The Heart of Hospice is dedicated to helping personal and professional caregivers, providing them with information and education so they can make informed choices in regard to hospice.

http://www.theheartofhospice.com/home

WOMEN IN-DEPTH
Listen in as Lourdes Viado PHD, MFT, talks with therapists, coaches, writers, and other experts about the inner lives of women: their struggles, fears, hopes, and dreams.

https://lourdesviado.com

END OF LIFE CARE

JANE BRODY'S GUIDE TO THE GREAT BEYOND
This New York Times columnist has a nice breezy style that covers what we should all think about before we get to the end of life.

FINAL GIFTS–*Understanding the Special Awareness, Needs, and Communications of the Dying* by Maggie Callanan and Patricia Kelley
Two hospice nurses share their intimate experiences with patients at the end of life, drawn from more than twenty years experience tending the terminally ill.

ON DEATH AND DYING by Elisabeth Kubler-Ross
In this famous classic, Kubler-Ross explores the five stages of grief through sample interviews and conversations.

PASSAGES IN CAREGIVING by Gail Sheehy
This is a Passages inspired book about the spiritual journey that we travel as caregivers. This is essentially a spiritual and emotional support book following Sheehy's years she spent caregiving for her husband.

THE TIBETAN BOOK OF LIVING AND DYING by Sogyal Rinpoche
A manual for life and death, and a great source of sacred inspiration from the heart of the Tibetan tradition.

THE FOUR THINGS THAT MATTER MOST by Ira Byock, MD .
This book deals with an important aspect of death: unresolved issues.

LIFE AFTER LIFE by Raymond A. Moody Jr., MD
One hundred people who have experienced "clinical death" and were revived, tell in their own words, what lies beyond death.

END OF LIFE CARE FOR THE ELDERLY

A BITTERSWEET SEASON—*Caring for Our Aging Parents and Ourselves* by Jane Gross
This book has that "I've-walked-in-your-moccasins" feeling and is just a great read. It is completely focused on care for an elderly parent.

HOW TO CARE FOR AGING PARENTS by Virginia Morris
This big book is packed with great information about eldercare.

GRIEF

HOW TO GO ON LIVING WHEN SOMEONE YOU LOVE DIES by Therese A. Rando
This comprehensive guide leads you gently through the painful but necessary process of grieving and helps you find the best way for yourself.

BOOKS FOR CHILDREN AND TEENS

WHEN DINOSAURS DIE—*A Guide to Understanding Death* by Laurie Krasny Brown and Marc Brown
This comprehensive guide lets children know that death is simply a part of life. It covers everything from deaths of pets, to deaths of close family members both young and old, and ways to memorialize all of them. It's a good book to have in the house before you need it.

THE FALL OF FREDDIE THE LEAF—*A Story of Life for All Ages,* by Leo Buscaglia
A warm, simple story about a leaf named Freddy, who goes through the changing of the seasons with his fellow leaves and learns about the delicate balance between life and death.

TEAR SOUP, *A Recipe of Healing After Loss* by Pat Schwiebert and Chuck DeKlyen
Beautifully illustrated book rich in wisdom and concrete recommendations on grief for adults and children to be shared for years to come.

HEALING YOUR GRIEVING HEART FOR TEENS—*100 Practical Ideas* by Alan D. Wolfelt, PhD
This book offers, with great sensitivity and insight, suggestions for healing activities that can help teens learn to express their grief and mourn naturally.

I WILL REMEMBER YOU by Laura Dower
An inspirational and accessible guide to coping with loss. It includes personal stories from teens, advice from a grief counselor, and dozens of hands-on creative exercises to help teens move through their grief.

THE GRIEVING TEEN: *A Guide for Teenagers and their Friends* by Helen Fitzgerald
This book discusses the difficult emotions and range of situations teens may find themselves in after a loss, including family changes, issues with friends, problems at school, and moving forward with one's life.

STRAIGHT TALK ABOUT DEATH FOR TEENAGERS: *How to Cope with Losing Someone You Love* by Earl Grollman
Offers straight from the heart information about the thoughts, feelings and questions teens might have when someone they care about dies.

YOU ARE NOT ALONE: *Teens Talk About Life After the Loss of a Parent* by Lynne Hughes
Grieving teens explain the way they dealt with the death of a parent. They discuss what helps, what doesn't, how to stay connected with the deceased, and how to begin healing.

INDEX

A

abdominal swelling 121
acceptance 4
achiness: general end-of-life achiness 95
active labor: one to two hours before death 145
acupuncture 135
acyclovir 127, 177
adjunctive drugs 135
adjuvant drugs 132,
adult disposable diapers 69, 75, 76, 81, 82, 111, 160
adult foster homes 42
advance directive 6, 12, 13, 20, 66
Advil 95, 98, 106, 126, 127, 132, 177, 178, 180
AFH 42. See also Adult Foster Homes
after death
  direct cremation 155
  funeral 14,16, 19,20, 144, 151-159, 168,
  green burial 155
  home burial 155
  memorial 19, 20, 153-159, 168
  scattering ashes 157
  wake 26, 140, 151, 156
  funeral arrangements 154
    burial (interment) 154
    cremation 154, 155
agitation 96, 101-103, 106, 113, 132, 144, 148, 178-180
AIDs 114
Aleve 95, 126, 132, 177
ALF 41. See also Assisted Living Facilities
ALS 66, 111, 120, 134, 173
alternative pain relief 134
Alzheimer's 41, 42, 45, 66, 101, 102, 106, 133, 178
anger 4
antibiotic 70, 98, 107, 109, 109, 121, 122, 173, 175, 179
Anticipatory Grief 5
anti-inflammatories 126, 127, 132, 133, 175, 177, 178
anxiety 18, 28, 64, 96, 99, 100, 106, 110, 113, 117, 119, 135, 173, 175-180
anxiety and agitation 95, 96
aromatherapy 135
artificial hydration 66
ascites 121, 173
aspirin 106, 173, 175
assessing pain 124
assisted living facilities 41
Atarax 114, 177
Ativan 96, 99, 100, 103, 106, 113, 117, 119, 121, 129, 130, 133, 144, 147, 148, 177
Atropine 100, 120, 128, 133, 147, 177
Aveeno 114

B

Baclofen 111, 133, 177
bargaining 4
bed bath 86
bedbound patient 21, 47, 69, 75, 82, 97, 112
bedpan 80, 81, 111
bed rails 59
bedside commode 54, 57, 60, 68, 75, 79, 111, 173, 177
bed sores 76, 83, 84, 87, 94, 97
belladonna 128, 133
Benadryl 114, 116, 120, 130, 133, 177
bladder spasms 94, 98
bleeding 66, 94, 98, 99
bone metastasis 126
bone pain 126
bowel obstruction 117
BRAT diet 107, 117
breathing difficulties 94, 100
burial (interment) 154
Butt Paste 85, 118

C

Caladryl lotion 127
Calmoseptine 85
Canasol 134, 177
cancer 4, 7, 32, 45, 49, 66, 70, 98, 102, 110, 111, 114, 116, 122, 126, 127, 134, 173, 174, 178
candida thrush 115
catheter 69, 70, 98, 112
  catheter cramping 98
cellulitis 121

Children
symptoms of grief 168
should children go to funerals 160
chronic pain 125
coma 145
semi-comatose 145
combativeness 94, 101
Compazine 64, 99, 117, 130, 177
complicated grief 166, 167. see also grief
condom catheter 69
confusion 58, 94, 102, 103, 106, 122, 131, 134
constipation 63, 66, 67, 94, 96, 104, 111, 131
cremation 154, 155

D

daily care log 64
death certificates 160
death: how do we know he is dead? 153
Decadron 112, 126, 132, 177
dementia 42, 96, 102, 106, 111
dementia at the end of life 106
denial 3
Depakote 103, 178
depression 4, 40, 106
Desitin 85, 118
Diarrhea and Cramps 107
Diflucan 114, 116, 118
Dilaudid 100, 129, 130, 178
direct cremation 155
disability office 36
Ditropan 98, 111, 178
diuretic 100, 174, 178
DME 57
DNR (Do Not Resuscitate.) 13
draw sheet 76, 77, 85, 9
Dr. Ira Byock 8
Ducolax 67, 104
durable medical equipment. see also dme
durable power of attorney 14
Duragesic (fentanyl) 130

E

early labor: two to four months before death 140
egg crate mattress pad 75
Elavil 114, 127, 132, 178
electric lift chair 58
Elisabeth Kubler-Ross 3
end of life visions 109
esophageal bleeding 99
ethical wills 8
extreme headache 119

F

Facing Fears . . .
of abandonment 7
of being a burden to family 7
of loss of dignity and losing control 6, 7
of no longer being useful 7
of pain and suffering 6
fallproof your home 54
fallproof bathrooms 54
false beliefs about pain 125
Famciclovir 127, 178
feeding guidelines 64
feeding tube 66, 141
fever 70, 94, 108, 130
fireproof your home 55
Five Stages of Grief 3
Five Wishes document 12
Flagyl powder 97
Fleets 105
Flomax 111, 178
fracture pan 80
funeral 14, 16, 19, 20, 144, 151, 153, 154, 155, 156, 157, 159, 168
funeral home 16, 19, 151, 153, 154, 155, 159
Furosemide 100

G

Gait belt 57
going to the toilet 68
green burial 155
grief , 5, 161, 163, 165, 166, 168
child's symptoms of grief 168
guardianship 14

H

Haldol 96, 101, 103, 106, 110, 113, 117, 133, 144, 178
hallucinations 94, 109, 110
hastening death 21
healthcare provider 93
health care representative 12
heart attack 119, 128
helper drugs 132
helping your confused loved one 104

hiccups 94, 110, 111
home burial 155
home health aids 44
home instead 36
hospice 4, 6, 8, 21, 24, 25, 32, 34, 37, 38, 41-49, 54, 57, 60, 93, 99, 119, 128, 131, 145, 150, 151, 160, 162
hospice chaplain 44
Hospice Foundation of America 49
Hospice Houses 42
hospice medical director 44
hospice team 44
hospital bed 58
hot or cold therapy 134
how do I help my children grieve 168
How to . . .
- **avoid** pressure sores 85
- change a diaper of a bedbound patient 82
- change the bed linens 90
- give a bath/shower 70
- give a bed bath 86
- give an enema 105
- move a patient in the bed 76
- turn patient onto her side 78

Hoyer Lift 60
hydrocortisone creams 114
hygiene 70

I
ibuprofen 113, 133, 175
Imodium 107, 178
important papers 16
incontinence 75, 94, 111, 117, 122
incontinent patient 68
in-dwelling catheter 112
insomnia 94, 112
internal bleeding 119, 128
itching 94, 113, 114, 118

J
jaundice 94, 114, 115
just before death 149

K
Keppra 119, 178
Klonipin 130
KY gel 105

L
Lactulose 103, 104, 178
Lasix 121, 130, 133, 147, 178
Legal Decisions
- will 15
- durable power of attorney 14
- guardianship 14
- legal guardian 13
- living trust 15
- trust 15

Levsin 128, 133, 178
Lidocaine 116, 120, 178
life insurance 7, 16, 158, 160
liquid morphine sulfate 129
living memorial 8
living trust 15, 160

M
Maalox 116, 120
male urinal 69
Marinol 134, 179
massage 228, 85, 97, 113, 135
medical marijuana (cannabis) 134
medical social worker 44
meditation and guided imagery 27, 135
memorial 19, 20, 153, 154, 156, 157, 159, 168
memory care units 42
memory loss 106
Metamucil 105
Methadone 130, 179
Miconazole 118, 179
Milk of Magnesia 104, 179
Miracle Mouthwash 116, 120
Miralax 67, 104, 179
morphine 6, 95, 96, 99-101, 113, 114, 119, 122, 126-132, 147, 148, 178-181
- fears about morphine 131
- morphine sulfate 129

mouth care 72
mouth sores 94, 115, 116
MS 98, 111, 129
MS Contin 129

N
Nabilone 134
narcotic pain medications 67
National Association of Professional Geriatric Care 39

National Hospice and Palliative Care Organization 39
nausea and vomiting 116
nebulizing treatments 100
nerve block 133
nerve pain 127
Neurontin 127, 132, 133, 179
Nitroglycerin 119, 133, 179
non-medical pain relief 134
non steroidal anti-inflammatories 132
NSAIDS 132
Norco 126, 179
nosebleeds 99
nursing homes 41
Nystatin 116, 118, 179

O

obituary 159
On Death and Dying 3
opioids 129, 130, 131, 132, 133, 134, 179
opioid side effects 130
opium 128, 133
organ and body donations 20
over the bed table 59
Oxycodone 100, 129, 130, 179
Oxycontin 130, 179
oxygen 31, 43, 55-57, 97, 101-103, 109, 113, 115, 119, 121, 147, 174, 175

P

Pain 3, 5-7, 11, 12, 17, 21, 24, 28, 43, 46-49, 63-67, 91-106, 112-135, 139, 145-148, 150, 167, 173, 175-181
assessing pain 124
bone pain 126
false beliefs about pain 125
nerve pain 127
pain control 129, 133, 134
signs of physical pain 124
somatic pain (general pain) 126
sudden, severe pain 128
four basic principles of good pain control 123
visceral pain (organ pain) 128
WHO pain ladder 181
alternative pain relief 134
medical marijuana (cannabis) 134
helper drugs 135

Pain (cont):
Morphine 131
nerve block 133
non-medical pain relief 134
aromatherapy 135
hot or cold therapy 134
massage 28, 85, 97, 113, 135
meditation and guided imagery 27, 135
palliative sedation 134
PLO (pluronic lecithin organogel 133
radiation 127, 134
specialists 135
acupuncture 135
reflexology 28, 135
synthetic opioids 129, 130
pain pump 129
palliative care v, 43, 49
palliative sedation 134
Pamelor 127, 179
Paracentesis 48, 122, 175
Parkinson's 120
patient's clothing 75
Paxil 114, 179
peripheral edema 121
peripheral neuropathy 114
physical therapists 45
physician's orders for life sustaining treatment 13
pillows 76
pleurx catheter 122
PLO (pluronic lecithin organogel 133
POA 13
POLST 13
power of attorney 13, 14
Prednisone 114, 118, 126, 132, 179
pressure sores 58, 61, 75, 81, 84, 85, 97
Prevacid 132, 179
Prilosec 132, 179
probate 14, 15
pyridium 98, 179

R

radiation 49, 66, 115, 118, 126, 134
rash 94, 117
red mottling 148
registered nurse case manager 44
Reglan 111, 117, 130, 179

regular bowel movements 67
Remeron 113, 180
right to die 21
Robinul 100, 120, 180

S

Sarna 114, 180
scattering ashes 157
Scopolamine 100, 120, 128, 14
seizures 94, 118, 119
semi-comatose 145
Senakot 104
senior services 36, 42
Senna S 67
Seroquel 96, 103, 106, 110, 113, 180
severe difficulty breathing 119
shingles 127
shower chair 60
signs of physical pain 124
skilled nursing facilities 41
skin sores 87
sleeping positions in bed 76
Sleepy Time Tea 113
Smooth Move Tea 67, 104
SNF 41. see also skilled nursing facilities
Social Security Administration 153, 154, 158, 160
soma 133, 180
somatic pain (general pain) 126
specialists 135
spiritual tools 26-29
steroids 128, 132
stroke 12, 81, 88, 119, 129, 173, 174, 175, 177
sudden changes in behavior 103
sudden severe pain 94, 119, 128
sundowning 102
swallowing difficulties/throat secretions 120
swelling 87, 121, 122, 128, 174
swelling in feet and legs, and belly 120
Symptoms and Solutions:
  achiness: general end-of-life 94
  bedsores or pressure sores 94, 97
  bladder spasms 94, 98
  bleeding 66, 94, 98, 99
Symptoms and Solutions(cont):
  breathing difficulties 94, 100
  combativeness 94, 101, 102
  confusion 94, 102, 103, 106
  constipation 63, 66, 67, 94, 96, 104, 111, 131
  diarrhea and cramps 107
  fever 70, 94, 108, 130
  hallucinations 94, 109, 110
    end of life visions 109
  hiccups 94, 110, 111
  incontinence 75, 94, 111
  insomnia 94, 112
  itching 94, 113, 114, 118
  jaundice 94, 114, 115
  mouth sores 994, 115, 116
  nausea and vomiting 117
    bowel obstruction 117
  nosebleeds 99
  rash 94, 117
  seizures 94, 119
  sudden severe pain 94, 119
    stroke 12, 81, 88, 119, 129, 173-177
    heart attack 119, 128
    internal bleeding 119, 128
    severe difficulty breathing 119
  swallowing difficulties/throat secretions 120
  swelling in feet and legs, and belly 120
    abdominal swelling 121
    sudden swelling in one leg 121
  urination: difficult and/or painful 122
    urinary tract infections (UTI) 98, 123

T

Tegretol 132
ten ways to decrease stress 32-36
the business of death 158-163
the caregiver's journey 5
the conversation 12-16
the emotional journey 3
the labor of death 140-150
the living trust 15
the moment of death 150
the spiritual journey 6
Thoracentesis 48, 100, 175
Thorazine 100, 101, 111, 180
Thrush 115
toileting a bedbound patient 79
  bedside commode 60, 79
  using a bedpan or fracture pan 80

toothette 72, 116, 120, 147- 149
Tophranil 114
trained hospice volunteers 45
transfer bench 60, 71
trapeze 59
travel metaphors 142, 144, 148
Trazadone 113
trust 14
trust accounts 160
tumor 128, 174
Tylenol 95, 106, 109, 126, 147, 177-180, 181

U

urinary tract infection (UTI) 101, 103, 106, 111, 122, 176
    Sudden Changes in Behavior 122, 176
Urination: Difficult and/or Painful 123

V

Valium 96, 119, 130, 133, 180
Versed 119, 134, 180
Veteran's Affairs Office (VA) 36, 41, 153, 154, 159, 160
Vicoden 113
visceral pain (organ pain) 128
viscous Lidocaine 116

W

wake 26, 140, 151, 156
walker 57
washing hair in bed 89
What does a funeral home do? 154
What do I do at the moment of death? 150
wheelchair 58
when to call 911 93
whole body donation 20
WHO pain ladder 181
Why won't they eat? 65
World Health Organization 181

X

Xanax 96, 103, 106, 113, 180

Z

Zantac 132, 180
Zeasorb 118
Zofran 99, 114, 117, 130, 180

ACKNOWLEDGMENTS

It takes a village to research, write, vet, and proof a guidebook of this scope. We'd like to thank all of the editors, doctors, nurses, and friends whose advice is carefully woven into this book. Special thanks to the following:

Katie Adkison, RN
Norma Beecham
Dan Brandenberg, MD
Nancy Brandenberg, RN
Stephen Brummer, MD
Sheila Burns
Kathy Bryon
Mary Clark, RN
Kris Earl, RN
Mark Flickinger
John Forsyth
Rebecca Gabriel
Wendy Gaffey, RN
Barbara Brownell Grogan
Susan Hearn
Malcolm Hillgartner
Michael J. Hume
Rebecca Hutchison, MD
Holly James, RN, WOSN
Gordon Javna
Katie Leonis, RN, MSN
Eric McFarland, MD
Maggie McLaughlin
Robin Miller, MD, MHS
Jaimie Muehlhausen
Carol Ortlip
Michele Ortlip
Robin Potochnick, LCSW
Deanna Rhoden, RPH
Vickie Roundy, RN, CHPN
Chris Tomasino
Diana Van Vleck
Jack Wiens
Linda B. White, MD

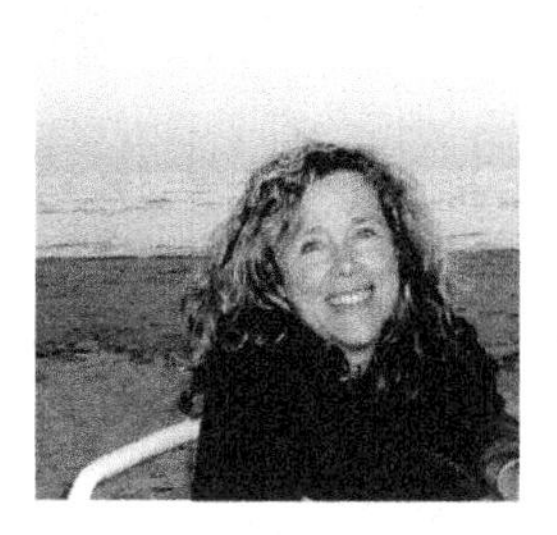

Katie Ortlip, LCSW, is a Hospice Expert on *SHARECARE,* Dr. Ahmet Oz's online health and wellness platform that provides consumers with expert information to help them lead healthier lives. Katie is co-author of *Spiritual Tools for the Dying,* a booklet distributed by Asante Health Care of Oregon to patients on hospice. She received her nursing degree from Santa Barbara City College in 1982 and then spent three years working in neonatology at St. Luke's-Roosevelt Hospital in New York City and Mary Dartmouth-Hitchcock Hospital in Hanover, New Hampshire. Katie then spent six years working in pediatrics at Albany Medical Center while earning a BA in Psychology and Masters of Social Work at SUNY-Albany. She moved to Ashland, Oregon, with her family in 1992, and has worked as a nurse and social worker for Asante Hospice for the past twenty-five years. During that time she has studied with Richard and Mary Groves of the Sacred Art of Living Center, completing the Sacred Art of Dying program. She has also studied with Frank Ostaseski, founding director of Zen Hospice Project in San Francisco. Katie has a special interest in ethics at the end of life, and has attended conferences with Ira Byock, Barbara Karnes and most recently the Kinsman Conference on Stewardship in Health Care.

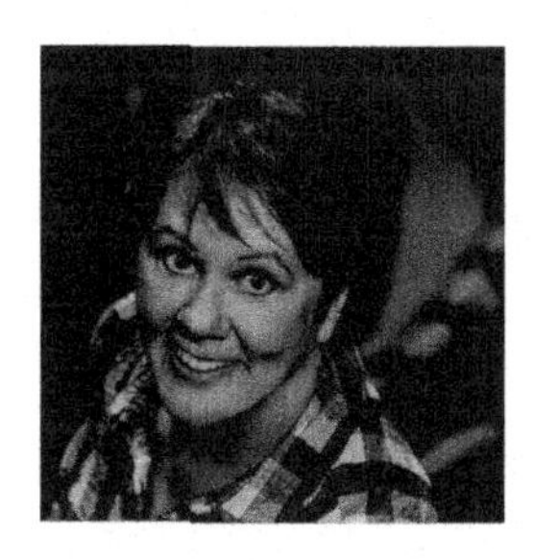

Jahnna Beecham most recently edited National Geographic's *Science Encyclopedia,* which was released in the fall of 2016, and was a contributing editor for National Geographic's *The Ultimate Explorer Field Guide: Birds.* For the past 15 years she has been a contributing writer and editor for *Uncle John's Bathroom Reader*—both the adult books and *For Kids Only.* Under the pen name Jahnna N. Malcolm, Jahnna Beecham and Malcolm Hillgartner have written more than 130 books for juveniles and young adults for Scholastic, Simon & Schuster, Random House, HarperCollins, Bantam and others. They wrote Scholastic's *The Baby-Sitters Club Guide to Babysitting,* working with doctors and childcare specialists. Jahnna has written award-winning learning systems and books for *Hooked on Phonics.* She also wrote a humorous parenting column for *Sesame Street Parents Magazine* and Children's Television Workshop online. Jahnna has directed audiobook recordings for Brilliance audio and with composer-lyricist Malcolm Hillgartner, has written *The Best Christmas Pageant Ever: the Musical*, published by Playscripts.

Notes and Important Numbers

Made in the USA
Middletown, DE
12 November 2020